Minimally Invasive Surgery - Transforming Care with Precision

Edited by Kunal Bhakhri
and Alessandro Maraschi

Published in London, United Kingdom

Minimally Invasive Surgery - Transforming Care with Precision
http://dx.doi.org/10.5772/intechopen.1008589
Edited by Kunal Bhakhri and Alessandro Maraschi

Contributors
Alessandro Maraschi, Bianca Sabrina Ribolzi, Dimitrios Balafoutas, Elias Tsakos, Emmanouil Xydias, Ettore Dalmasso, Giovanni Busacca, Ivano Morra, Krit Vikan, Luciano Ola, Nikolaos Vlahos, Padungkiat Tangpiroontham, Ralf Joukhadar, Ömer Faruk Sağlam

First published in London, United Kingdom, 2026 by IntechOpen
IntechOpen is the global imprint of INTECHOPEN LIMITED, registered in England and Wales, registration number: 11086078, 167-169 Great Portland Street, London, W1W 5PF, United Kingdom

For EU product safety concerns: IN TECH d.o.o., Prolaz Marije Krucifikse Kozulić 3, 51000 Rijeka, Croatia, info@intechopen.com or visit our website at intechopen.com.

British Library Cataloguing-in-Publication Data
A catalogue record for this book is available from the British Library

Minimally Invasive Surgery - Transforming Care with Precision
Edited by Kunal Bhakhri and Alessandro Maraschi
p. cm.
Print ISBN 978-1-83634-827-6
Online ISBN 978-1-83634-826-9
eBook (PDF) ISBN 978-1-83634-828-3

Meet the editors

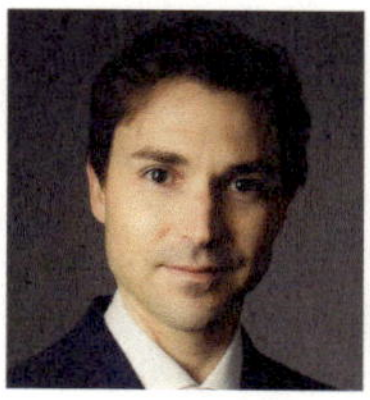

Alessandro Maraschi is a Consultant Thoracic Surgeon at University College London Hospitals (UCLH), specializing in minimally invasive and robotic thoracic surgery. He trained across leading European centers and has developed expertise in VATS, RATS, and complex lung and mediastinal procedures. His clinical practice integrates advanced imaging, enhanced recovery pathways, and a strong focus on surgical precision and patient-centered care. Mr. Maraschi is actively involved in research, education, and international collaboration, and his work spans robotic innovation, perioperative optimization, and modern thoracic surgical strategies. He has authored multiple publications and serves as an Academic Editor with IntechOpen, contributing to the dissemination of contemporary surgical knowledge.

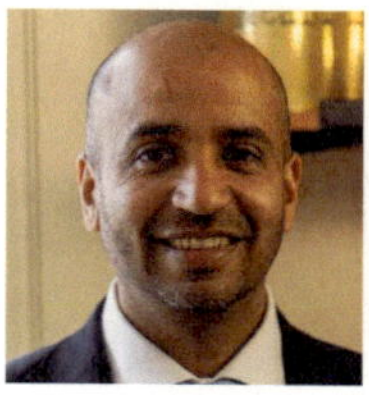

Kunal Bhakhri is Lead for Robotic and Minimal Access Thoracic Surgery at University College London Hospital, where he directs a nationally recognised, high-volume robotic thoracic programme. He has transformed service delivery by reducing postoperative length of stay to well below national benchmarks and expanding robotic case volume by 300% through strategic recruitment, mentoring, and workflow optimisation. As an academic surgeon, his work spans robotic innovation, chest wall conditions, surgical education, and system-level quality improvement. He has advised national commissioning through the Thoracic Surgery Clinical Reference Group, secured significant regional and national funding, and led the establishment of the Chest Wall Database. A strong advocate for education, he has developed widely used e-learning modules, serves as a Royal College Tutor, and proctors robotic surgeons across Europe. His research contributions include soft-robotic ventilatory technologies, digital education, cost-effectiveness of robotic surgery, 3D surgical modelling, and future AI-integrated thoracic practice.

Contents

Preface

Minimally invasive surgery has become one of the most significant transformations in modern operative care. Over the last three decades, advances in optics, instrumentation, anesthesia, and digital technology have not only refined surgical precision but also redefined what is considered achievable within each specialty. The shift from large incisions to smaller, targeted access routes has reshaped patient experiences and clinical outcomes, promoting faster recovery, reduced pain, and enhanced perioperative safety. What began as a technological evolution has now matured into a global standard of excellence, one that continues to expand as robotics, artificial intelligence, and advanced imaging tools accelerate the boundaries of innovation.

The ambition of this volume is to provide a multidisciplinary perspective on the development, adoption, and refinement of minimally invasive techniques across different surgical specialties.

The book brings together both broad overviews and highly specialized insights, highlighting not only where minimally invasive surgery stands today but also where it is heading as we enter a new phase of integration between digital and operative practice.

The volume opens with *Introductory Chapter: Minimally Invasive Surgery: Contemporary Evidence, System Integration, and Future Directions*, which provides an overview of the current state of minimally invasive surgery and the factors influencing its implementation in clinical practice. The chapter introduces key themes that recur throughout the book, including evidence, training, and system integration, and sets the scene for the specialty-focused chapters that follow.

The central section of the volume explores the application of minimally invasive approaches within urology and gynecology. In *Retroperitoneal Laparoscopic Nephrectomy for the Management of Polycystic Kidney Disease*, the authors offer a detailed overview of retroperitoneal access, highlighting how minimally invasive techniques can be effectively applied even in complex renal pathology, where anatomical distortion poses significant technical challenges. In parallel, *Current Surgical Treatment of Endometrial Carcinoma: The Role of Robotic Surgery* examines how robotic systems have refined oncologic gynecologic surgery. Through enhanced dexterity, 3D visualization, and improved ergonomics, robotic platforms have supported more precise dissection and staging, representing a substantial evolution within this specialty.

The final section of the book focuses on minimally invasive thoracic surgery. *Evolution of Minimally Invasive Thoracic Surgery* traces the significant milestones in the development of both VATS and RATS approaches, outlining how they have reshaped thoracic practice by enabling complex pulmonary and mediastinal procedures to be performed with decreasing invasiveness. The concluding chapter, *Robotic*

Subxiphoid Thymectomy: Approaches and Techniques, provides a focused analysis of robotic access to the anterior mediastinum. The subxiphoid route, which offers superior visualization and bilateral access, is explored in detail, underscoring the continued refinement of techniques within robotic thoracic surgery.

Across all chapters, a unifying theme emerges: minimally invasive surgery is no longer defined solely by smaller incisions, but by the integration of technology, precision, and multidisciplinary collaboration. The evolution of these techniques has required cooperation between surgeons, anesthetists, engineers, computer scientists, and perioperative specialists. It has also relied on rigorous training, continuous evaluation of outcomes, and the willingness of clinicians to adapt to new methods while maintaining patient safety at the center of practice.

We hope that this volume serves as a resource for clinicians, trainees, researchers, and all professionals engaged in advancing minimally invasive surgery. By presenting a broad yet cohesive overview of developments across specialties, the book aims to foster reflection, support clinical decision-making, and inspire continued innovation. Minimally invasive surgery remains a field in motion, and its future will depend on our collective ability to learn from each other, integrate new technologies responsibly, and maintain a commitment to excellence throughout the surgical journey.

I extend my sincere gratitude to all contributing authors for their expertise, dedication, and collaborative spirit. Their work reflects the strength of multidisciplinary cooperation and the shared ambition to advance the quality of surgical care worldwide.

Alessandro Maraschi MD, FRCS
Thoracic Surgery,
University College London Hospitals (UCLH),
London, United Kingdom

Dr. Kunal Bhakhri
University College London Hospitals NHS Foundation Trust,
London, UK

Section 1

Innovations in Minimally Invasive Surgery

Chapter 1

Introductory Chapter: Minimally Invasive Surgery – Contemporary Evidence, System Integration and Future Directions

Alessandro Maraschi

1. Introduction

Minimally invasive surgery (MIS) emerged as a pragmatic response to a problem that surgeons have long recognised – the burden imposed not only by the disease itself but also by the way it is accessed. Traditional open approaches, while effective in achieving anatomical and oncological goals, are intrinsically associated with tissue trauma, postoperative pain, delayed mobilisation, and prolonged recovery. The early development of laparoscopic and thoracoscopic techniques was, therefore, driven by a clinical need to reduce access-related morbidity while preserving or improving procedural effectiveness.

As minimally invasive techniques became more widely adopted, their benefits extended beyond immediate postoperative outcomes. Reduced surgical trauma translated into earlier mobilisation, fewer wound-related complications, and more predictable recovery trajectories. Over time, these advantages altered the balance between therapeutic benefit and treatment burden, influencing not only individual patient outcomes but also broader patterns of healthcare utilisation. Large observational analyses have documented the progressive replacement of open surgery with minimally invasive approaches across multiple procedures, reflecting a shift from innovation to consolidation within routine practice [1].

Importantly, the expansion of MIS has not been uniform or indiscriminate. Its adoption has varied according to procedure complexity, institutional expertise, and available infrastructure. Open surgery remains essential in specific clinical contexts, including advanced disease, complex anatomy, and emergency settings. Contemporary surgical practice, therefore, reflects a mature equilibrium in which minimally invasive and open approaches coexist, guided by patient factors, disease characteristics, and system capability rather than ideology alone [2].

2. Evidence and Clinical Outcomes

With wider adoption of MIS, the evidence base has become increasingly focused on comparative effectiveness and long-term outcomes. Beyond short-term recovery metrics, recent studies increasingly address long-term oncological and patient-centred outcomes. In thoracic surgery, comparative analyses have demonstrated that robot-assisted and video-assisted lobectomy for non-small cell lung cancer achieve equivalent long-term oncological outcomes, including disease-free and overall survival, with no compromise in nodal staging [3]. These findings support the oncologic reliability of minimally invasive lung resection when applied within appropriately structured programmes.

Further insight into the real-world applicability of MIS comes from studies focusing on complex patient cohorts. Multicentre data examining outcomes in obese patients undergoing lung cancer surgery have shown that minimally invasive approaches, including both robotic and video-assisted techniques, can be safely applied in higher-risk populations, with acceptable perioperative and oncological outcomes when compared with open surgery [4]. Such evidence reinforces the notion that the value of MIS lies not only in idealised settings but also in its capacity to address surgical complexity when supported by appropriate expertise.

Patient-reported outcomes provide an additional dimension to the evaluation of MIS. Comparative analyses of quality of life following robotic, video-assisted, and open lung cancer surgery demonstrate that minimally invasive approaches are associated with earlier recovery of physical function and improved short- to mid-term quality-of-life measures [5]. These data highlight the importance of outcomes that extend beyond length of stay and complication rates, aligning surgical success more closely with patient experience and functional recovery.

3. Technology, Systems, and Implementation

Technological innovation has played a central role in enabling this evolution. Robotic platforms have addressed several limitations of conventional laparoscopy, offering enhanced dexterity, stable three-dimensional visualisation, and improved ergonomics. While superiority over conventional minimally invasive techniques is procedure-dependent, population-level analyses indicate that the introduction of robotic platforms has expanded the use of MIS rather than simply replacing existing techniques, creating a broader impact on access and service delivery [6].

The introduction of advanced technology has shifted MIS from a purely technical choice to a model that depends on imaging, perioperative pathways, and organisational structure [7]. As technology becomes more sophisticated, the importance of structured training, designated pathways, and outcome monitoring increases, particularly in relation to medico-legal responsibility and patient safety.

MIS has also driven changes in perioperative care. Enhanced recovery principles have evolved alongside reduced-access techniques, reinforcing their benefits through multimodal analgesia, early mobilisation, and standardised postoperative pathways. Evidence from large cohort analyses demonstrates that adherence to enhanced recovery protocols is associated with improved outcomes and reduced resource utilisation, underscoring the interdependence between surgical approach and perioperative system design [8].

4. Limitations and Future Directions

Despite its widespread adoption, MIS is not without limitations. Outcomes remain closely linked to experience, case volume, and the organisational context in which techniques are introduced. Learning curves are procedure-specific and can be prolonged, particularly when new platforms or technologies are adopted without structured training or adequate institutional support. In such settings, the theoretical advantages of minimally invasive approaches may be diluted or lost altogether.

Variability between centres remains a relevant issue. Differences in infrastructure, access to technology, team familiarity, and perioperative pathways continue to influence results, even when similar procedures are performed. This variability highlights an important distinction between technical feasibility and reproducibility. The ability to perform a minimally invasive operation does not, in itself, guarantee consistent outcomes across different environments.

These considerations reinforce the need to view MIS within a broader framework of service design rather than as an isolated technical solution. Programme development, case selection, data monitoring, and governance play a critical role in determining whether minimally invasive approaches translate into durable clinical benefits. Without this structure, expansion risks prioritising access over quality, with potential consequences for both outcomes and training.

The current challenge for MIS is no longer technical feasibility but consistency. Outside high-volume centres, the key question is whether minimally invasive results can be reproduced consistently in routine practice. This requires structured training, appropriate case selection, and institutional frameworks capable of supporting complex minimally invasive programmes over time. In this setting, MIS should be understood as an established approach whose value depends on how it is implemented, monitored, and sustained, rather than on continued technological novelty.

Acknowledgments

The author acknowledges the use of ChatGPT (OpenAI) for language polishing and editing in the chapter. No AI tools were used for data analysis or figure generation.

Author details

Alessandro Maraschi
Thoracic Surgery Department, University College London Hospitals NHS Foundation Trust, UK

*Address all correspondence to: alessandro.maraschi@gmail.com

References

[1] St John A, Caturegli I, Kubicki NS, Kavic SM. The Rise of Minimally Invasive Surgery: 16 Year Analysis of the Progressive Replacement of Open Surgery with Laparoscopy. JSLS : Journal of the Society of Laparoscopic & Robotic Surgeons. 2020;**24**(4): e202000076. DOI: 10.4293/JSLS.2020.00076

[2] Zhao Z, Gu J. Open surgery in the era of minimally invasive surgery. Chinese Journal of Cancer Research. 2022;**34**(1):63–65. DOI: 10.21147/j.issn.1000-9604.2022.01.06

[3] Fabbri G, Femia F, Lampridis S, Farinelli E, Maraschi A, Routledge T, Bille A. Long-Term Oncologic Outcomes in Robot-Assisted and Video-Assisted Lobectomies for Non-Small Cell Lung Cancer. Journal of Clinical Medicine. 2023;**12**(20):6609. DOI: 10.3390/jcm12206609

[4] Fabbri G, Femia F, Guerrera F, Della Beffa E, Farinelli E, Maraschi A, Lyberis P, Ruffini E, Billè A. Non-small cell lung cancer in obese patients: comparison of open, robotic and videothoracoscopic surgery. Journal of Thoracic Oncology. 2023. DOI: 10.1016/j.jtho.2023.09.1000

[5] Asemota N, Maraschi A, Lampridis S, Pilling J, King J, Le Reun C, Billè A. Comparison of quality of life after robotic, video-assisted, and open surgery for lung cancer. Journal of Clinical Medicine. 2023;**12**:6230. DOI: 10.3390/jcm12196230

[6] Sheetz KH, Claflin J, Dimick JB. Trends in the Adoption of Robotic Surgery for Common Surgical Procedures. JAMA Network Open. 2020;**3**(1):e1918911. DOI: 10.1001/jamanetworkopen.2019.18911

[7] Maraschi A, Fraccalini T, Bhakhri K. Robotic innovations in thoracic surgery: state of the art and future perspectives. In: Surgical Techniques and Procedures. IntechOpen; 2025. DOI: 10.5772/intechopen.1009163

[8] Sauro KM, Smith C, Ibadin S, et al. Enhanced Recovery After Surgery Guidelines and Hospital Length of Stay, Readmission, Complications, and Mortality: A Meta-Analysis of Randomized Clinical Trials. JAMA Network Open. 2024;**7**(6):e2417310. DOI: 10.1001/jamanetworkopen.2024.17310

Section 2

Minimally Invasive Techniques Across Surgical Specialties

Chapter 2

Retroperitoneal Laparoscopic Nephrectomy for the Management of Polycystic Kidney Disease

Giovanni Busacca, Ivano Morra, Luciano Ola, Bianca Sabrina Ribolzi and Ettore Dalmasso

Abstract

Laparoscopic nephrectomy has become an important surgical strategy in the management of symptomatic autosomal dominant polycystic kidney disease (ADPKD). Indications include chronic pain, recurrent cyst infections, hematuria, early satiety, or respiratory compromise due to massive renal enlargement, and space optimization prior to kidney transplantation. While the transperitoneal approach is more commonly used due to the larger working space it provides, the retroperitoneal approach offers specific advantages in selected cases. Notably, retroperitoneal access avoids intraperitoneal organ manipulation, reducing the risk of bowel injury and postoperative ileus, and is particularly beneficial in patients with a history of previous abdominal surgery. Despite the limited working space and technical difficulty posed by the large size of polycystic kidneys, experienced surgeons can achieve excellent outcomes with retroperitoneal laparoscopic nephrectomy. This approach minimizes peritoneal contamination in infected or hemorrhagic cysts and allows for a direct route to the renal hilum. In expert hands, retroperitoneal laparoscopic nephrectomy is a safe and effective option that contributes to reduced morbidity and faster recovery.

Keywords: polycystic kidney, minimally invasive approach, retroperitoneal surgery, laparoscopic renal surgery, End-stage renal disease

1. Introduction

Autosomal dominant polycystic kidney disease (ADPKD) is a significant hereditary condition worldwide, representing a major cause of kidney failure and ranking fourth among the indications for renal replacement therapy [1].

ADPKD comprises a group of dominantly inherited disorders associated with kidney cysts and extrarenal manifestations. The two major genes implicated in ADPKD are *PKD1* and *PKD2*, which together account for over 90% of genetically confirmed familial cases.

Renal involvement typically includes early-onset hypertension, chronic kidney pain, and progressive renal insufficiency. Extrarenal features may involve hepatic, splenic, and pulmonary cysts, as well as intracranial aneurysms – particularly Berry aneurysms of the circle of Willis – which are responsible for sudden death in approximately 8%–11% of affected individuals [2, 3]. Furthermore, nearly 50% of patients progress to end-stage kidney disease (ESKD) by the age of 60 [4].

Renal cyst formation in ADPKD leads to pathological kidney enlargement, progressively disrupting normal renal architecture and function. As the kidneys enlarge, patients may experience abdominal crowding, distension, or discomfort, often accompanied by nausea, early satiety, and chronic lower back pain. In addition, complications such as hypertension, recurrent pyelonephritis, nephrolithiasis, and episodes of gross hematuria are common and can significantly impair quality of life. In some cases, kidney volume increases to such an extent that there is insufficient space in the abdomen or pelvis to accommodate a renal allograft, thus complicating or precluding kidney transplantation. Nephrectomy is typically reserved for symptomatic cases, accounting for approximately 20% of patients, or to create space in anticipation of kidney transplantation.

When the kidneys retain residual urine output, surgery is usually delayed for as long as possible in order to preserve diuresis and avoid the decline in quality of life commonly observed in anuric patients undergoing dialysis [5].

The traditional approach historically described is open nephrectomy, performed through various surgical incisions such as subcostal or xiphopubic. However, these procedures are often associated with a high complication rate, with morbidity reaching up to 38% and a reported mortality rate of approximately 3% [6, 7].

Since the first reported application of laparoscopic techniques for the management of polycystic kidney disease, multiple studies have confirmed the feasibility and safety of this minimally invasive approach.

From a surgical perspective, the laparoscopic approach can be performed via the transperitoneal route, hand-assisted technique, or retroperitoneal access. Although the retroperitoneal approach is often overlooked due to the limited anatomical space – especially in cases of markedly enlarged polycystic kidneys – it actually represents a valid and effective option for treating this condition.

The following sections will describe the surgical technique and present data from our experience with patients affected by ADPKD who underwent laparoscopic nephrectomy via the retroperitoneal approach.

2. Surgery

Patients with polycystic kidney disease require a carefully structured multidisciplinary approach, in which close collaboration between the urologist and nephrologist is essential. These patients often come for urological evaluation at the stage of end-stage renal disease and are already on dialysis, with the goal of undergoing a "cleansing" nephrectomy in preparation for kidney transplantation. In patients presenting with gross hematuria or flank pain, contrast-enhanced abdominal CT should be performed to rule out active bleeding, suspicious renal lesions, or obstructive nephrolithiasis. In cases of suspected infected cysts, antibiotic therapy remains the first-line treatment. However, in the presence of recurrent

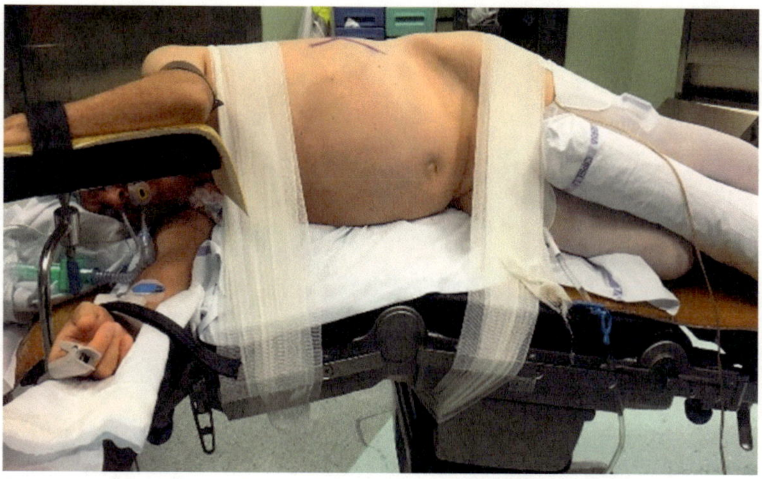

Figure 1.
Patient positioning.

pyelonephritis, large abscessed cysts, persistent gross hematuria, or chronic pain, surgical intervention becomes necessary to resolve the clinical condition effectively.

In the event of a positive urine culture, targeted antibiotic therapy is initiated based on the results of the antimicrobial susceptibility test.

Antibiotic prophylaxis is administered with 2 g of cefazolin intravenously one hour prior to the procedure. In patients with a documented allergy to penicillins or cephalosporins, clindamycin 600 mg IV is used as an alternative.

The patient is placed in a full flank position with slight table flexion at the level of the umbilical scar (**Figure 1**). A Foley catheter is routinely inserted unless the patient is anuric. The surgical field is then prepared under sterile conditions.

Retroperitoneal access is obtained via blunt dissection at the center of Petit's triangle. The access site is identified by locating anatomical landmarks: the tip of the 11th rib cranially, the iliac crest caudally, and the paravertebral muscles posteriorly. At the midpoint of an imaginary line connecting the 11th rib to the iliac crest lies a point of least resistance – corresponding to the center of Petit's triangle. At this location, a 1.5 cm skin incision is made with a scalpel, followed by blunt access to the retroperitoneal space. A Hasson trocar is subsequently placed at this site. Digital dissection is used to separate the fascial planes. A Gaur balloon dissector is then inserted to create a working space within the retroperitoneum; this step may be performed under direct vision using the laparoscopic optic.

Once the space is established, trocars are placed in a diamond-shaped configuration:

- A 10 mm trocar is placed approximately 4–6 cm laterally and 2 cm cranially to the initial incision.
- A 5 mm trocar is inserted approximately 4–6 cm medially and 2 cm cranially to the initial incision.
- Another 5 mm trocar is positioned just inferior to the tip of the 11th rib.

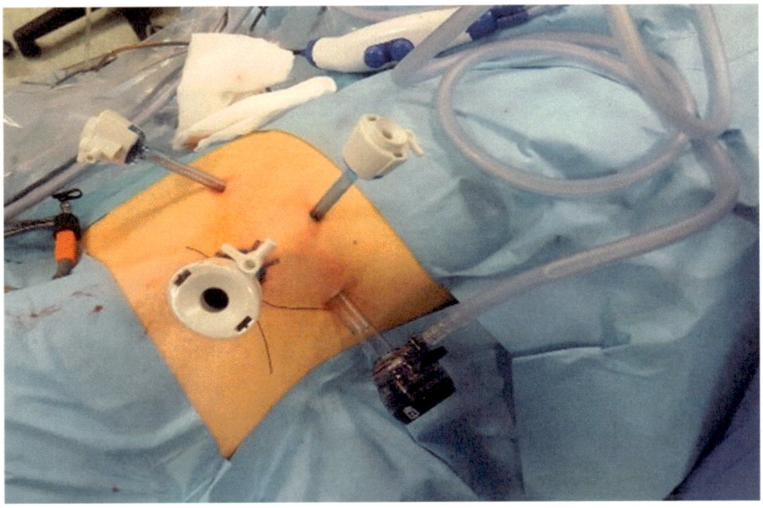

Figure 2.
Trocar placement.

The trocar configuration described refers to a surgical procedure on the left kidney (**Figure 2**). For right-sided procedures, the 10 mm trocar is positioned medially (to align with the dominant hand of a right-handed surgeon), while the 5 mm trocar is placed laterally. Once the Hasson trocar is secured, the retroperitoneal space is insufflated to a pressure of 12 mmHg.

Once the trocars are placed, the assistant surgeon introduces a 0° laparoscope through the Hasson trocar. The primary surgeon operates using the 10 and 5 mm trocars positioned cranially and laterally to the Hasson port. Through the 10 mm trocar, a suction device, bipolar forceps, or Hem-o-lok clip applier may be used, while the 5 mm port is typically used for forceps or an additional suction device. A second assistant may utilize the 5 mm trocar located just caudal to the tip of the 11th rib. The first critical anatomical landmark is the belly of the psoas muscle, which serves as a key orientation point in retroperitoneal surgery – especially when managing large renal masses. After identifying the psoas, the renal hilum is immediately sought to enable early and direct control of the vascular pedicle. In cases where the kidney is significantly enlarged and mobilization is impaired, a Chiba needle is inserted under direct laparoscopic visualization to aspirate the largest cysts. When this is necessary, the renal capsule is incised early to allow for full decompression. Otherwise, the renal capsule is opened only at the end of the procedure, either to facilitate cyst drainage or for specimen morcellation. Aspirated cyst fluid is routinely sent for microbiological culture to guide postoperative antibiotic therapy in case of infection-related complications. One of the main advantages of the retroperitoneal approach, especially in the hands of an experienced surgeon, is the possibility of direct and early access to the renal hilum. The renal artery and vein are secured and divided using Hem-o-lok clips (typically two clips on the vascular side of both artery and vein). Dissection proceeds caudally to identify the ureter, which is then followed to locate the gonadal vein. Both the ureter and gonadal vein are clipped with Hem-o-lok clips and divided. Dissection continues superiorly with the aim, when possible, of developing the plane between the kidney

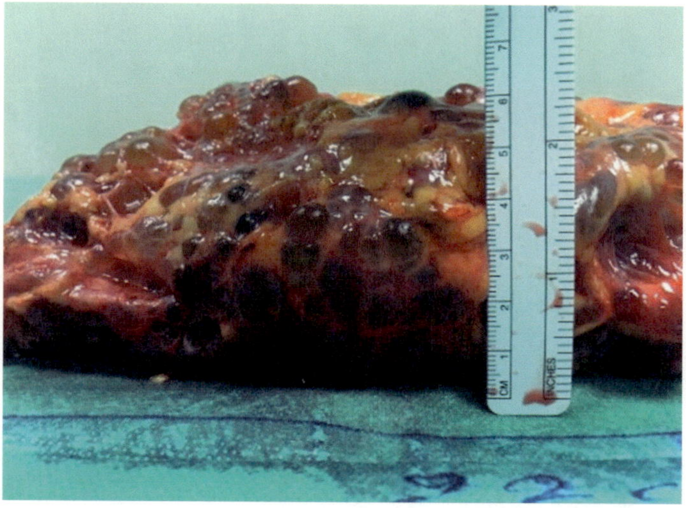

Figure 3.
Surgical specimen.

and adrenal gland in order to preserve the adrenal gland. However, due to the size of the kidney and/or inflammatory or infectious processes related to the cysts, perirenal and surrounding adipose tissue may be densely adherent, making adrenal sparing technically difficult or unsafe. In such cases, adrenalectomy is performed to minimize the risk of postoperative bleeding. Even when the renal size does not severely hinder the dissection, cyst aspiration is often performed at the end of the procedure to ease specimen extraction and reduce the size of the surgical incision. Once the upper pole is fully mobilized – whether or not the adrenal gland is preserved – dissection proceeds along the anterior surface of the kidney. The posterior parietal peritoneum may be densely adherent to the perirenal tissue due to prior cyst-related inflammatory or infectious processes. Particular caution is required during dissection to avoid injury to adjacent structures that may be at risk in this context, such as the duodenum, inferior vena cava (on the right), and pancreatic tail (on the left). Once the kidney has been fully mobilized, specimen morcellation may be performed, depending on its size, to reduce postoperative pain and minimize the cosmetic impact of the incision. In our experience, morcellation was required in only one case, using laparoscopic scissors, due to a particularly large renal volume of 5,400 cc. The surgical specimen (**Figure 3–4**) is placed in an endobag. For specimen removal, the incision at the Hasson trocar site is extended medially and caudally.

3. Discussion

In patients with ADPKD, symptomatic kidney enlargement and associated complications often necessitate the surgical removal of the native kidneys. In this context, laparoscopic nephrectomy has emerged as a minimally invasive alternative to open surgery, offering favorable perioperative outcomes and reduced morbidity. While the transperitoneal route has traditionally been the

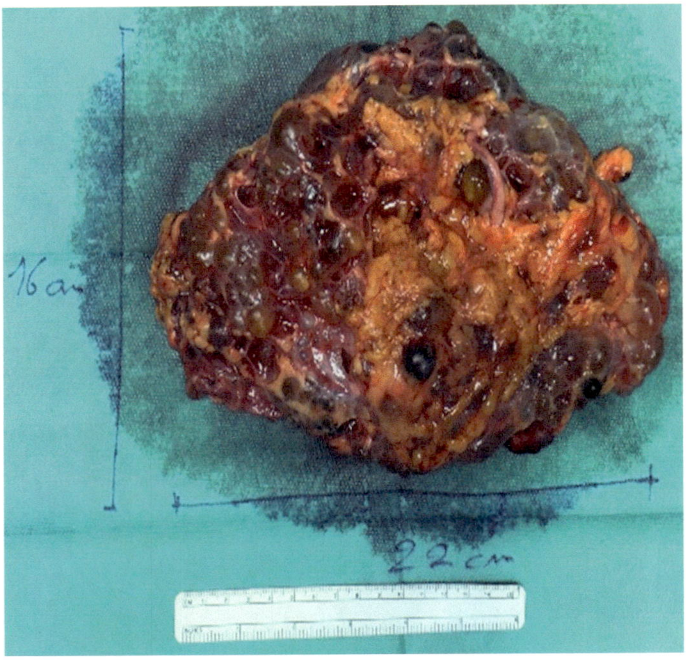

Figure 4.
Surgical specimen.

most commonly employed laparoscopic technique, the retroperitoneal approach offers several distinct advantages. By avoiding entry into the peritoneal cavity, this technique minimizes bowel manipulation, reduces the risk of postoperative ileus, and lowers the incidence of intraperitoneal adhesions – benefits particularly relevant in transplant candidates and those with prior abdominal surgeries (**Table 1**) [8–10].

One of the key concerns in laparoscopic nephrectomy for ADPKD is the technical complexity posed by the large kidney volume. Intraoperative decompression of cysts often facilitates dissection and mobilization, allowing for safer and more efficient extraction. While transperitoneal access provides a larger operative field, the retroperitoneal approach offers a more direct route to the renal hilum and avoids manipulation of intra-abdominal organs.

Approach	Main advantages	Main limitations
Open	Direct access, complete specimen removal	Morbidity, greater postoperative pain, longer recovery time
Transperitoneal	Wide operative field	Risk of intra-abdominal complications, adhesions
Retroperitoneal/ HALN	Less blood loss, shorter hospital stay, preservation of the peritoneum, better postoperative quality of life	Requires experience, limited working space, steep learning curve

Table 1.
Characteristics of the surgical approaches.

Recent literature has confirmed the safety and feasibility of the laparoscopic approach even in cases involving significantly enlarged polycystic kidneys. A systematic review and meta-analysis by Guo et al. demonstrated that laparoscopic nephrectomy, compared to the open technique, is associated with decreased blood loss, shorter hospital stays, fewer complications, and lower transfusion requirements, albeit with slightly longer operative times [6]. This is especially advantageous in patients preparing for transplantation, where minimizing allogeneic transfusion is crucial to reduce the risk of HLA sensitization [11]. Notably, Wyler et al. [9] reported a low complication rate and minimal blood loss in their initial experience with retroperitoneoscopic nephrectomy, confirming the technical feasibility of this approach even in the context of voluminous polycystic kidneys.

Chen et al. [12] evaluated predictors and outcomes in laparoscopic nephrectomy for ADPKD and confirmed that the minimally invasive approach is safe and effective, even in patients with massive kidney volumes. Their data demonstrated significantly reduced intraoperative blood loss and shorter hospitalization times compared to open surgery, with no increase in complication rates.

The retroperitoneal laparoscopic approach has been successfully applied to patients with massive renal volumes, yielding encouraging perioperative outcomes. Lyu et al. [11], in a comparative analysis between retroperitoneal laparoscopy and open nephrectomy in transplant candidates, observed superior outcomes in the laparoscopic group in terms of intraoperative bleeding, bowel recovery, and postoperative length of stay, despite slightly longer operative durations.

Preserving peritoneal integrity is particularly critical in patients undergoing or having undergone renal transplantation, as it facilitates access for graft placement and reduces the risk of adhesions that may complicate future surgical interventions. Kikkawa et al. [8] demonstrated the utility of the retroperitoneal approach in a transplanted patient, reporting no intraoperative or postoperative complications, supporting its safety and practicality in complex cases. Similarly, the approach is advantageous in dialysis-dependent patients, especially those utilizing peritoneal dialysis, by minimizing disruption of the peritoneal membrane [13].

Benoit et al. [14] directly compared the transperitoneal and retroperitoneal approaches in laparoscopic nephrectomy for polycystic kidney disease. In their study, there was no difference in terms of total complication rate and transfusion rate between the two groups; however, longer hospital stays and increased operative times were observed in the group undergoing retroperitoneal surgery. These findings appear to be influenced by complications experienced in a subset of retroperitoneal cases and by the lower overall surgical experience with the retroperitoneal approach. Operative times, however, do not appear to differ significantly after the first 20 cases of experience [14].

Management of large polycystic kidneys poses technical challenges, particularly during dissection and extraction. Intraoperative decompression of cysts is frequently necessary to facilitate mobilization. While some authors advocate the use of a morcellator to reduce incision size during specimen retrieval, caution must be exercised to prevent spillage of cystic contents, especially in the presence of infection or potential malignancy [15, 16]. Controlled aspiration under direct vision and the use of endobags can mitigate such risks, ensuring oncologic safety and minimizing contamination.

Despite its advantages, the retroperitoneal technique has inherent limitations. The confined working space and distorted anatomy due to cystic enlargement may complicate visualization and dissection. Furthermore, the learning curve for retroperitoneal laparoscopy is steeper compared to the transperitoneal route, requiring advanced laparoscopic skills and thorough anatomical knowledge [17, 18]. Therefore, proper patient selection and preoperative imaging to assess renal volume and anatomical landmarks are essential for procedural success.

It is important to note that the current evidence base consists predominantly of retrospective studies and case series, often from single institutions with relatively small sample sizes. There is a paucity of prospective, randomized trials directly comparing retroperitoneal and transperitoneal laparoscopic approaches or comparing laparoscopic versus open surgery in the ADPKD population.

Future research should aim to standardize surgical protocols, stratify patients based on renal volume and symptom burden, and assess long-term outcomes, including quality of life, postoperative recovery, impact on transplantation timelines, and cost-effectiveness. Multicenter, prospective trials will be essential to validate current findings and guide clinical decision-making.

4. Our experience

A total of 18 patients underwent nephrectomy for ADPKD in our department between January 2020 and March 2025. The main indication for surgery was to create space before renal transplantation (13 cases), while flank pain (3 cases) and hematuria (2 cases) were less common indications. Sixteen patients were on dialysis, including 13 on hemodialysis and 3 on peritoneal dialysis. The median Charlson Comorbidity Index was 4 (range: 4–5), and the mean hemoglobin level was 11.3 g/dL ± 1.4. The mean renal volume on CT scan was 2,870 cc (range: 1,080–5,400).

No conversion to open surgery was required, and no intraoperative complications were recorded. The mean operative time was 149 minutes (range 116–174). The mean cyst suction volume was 1,290 cc (range: 500–2,500), while the mean final renal volume was 810 cc (range: 477–1,164). The mean incision length was 7.3 cm (range: 7–8). The first passage of flatus occurred on postoperative day (POD) 1 in all cases, while the first stool was passed on POD 3 (range: 2–4).

The mean highest VAS pain score was 2.8 (range: 1–5) on POD 1, 2.8 (range: 2–5) on POD 2, and 2.3 (range: 1–5) on POD 3. The mean hemoglobin drop was 2.5 g/dL. Two patients experienced a complication graded higher than II according to the Clavien-Dindo classification (development of an arteriovenous fistula). Four patients required transfusion of one unit of red blood cells. No infectious complications occurred. The median hospital stay was 6 days (range: 3–9), and no complications were recorded within the first 30 days after surgery (**Table 2**).

5. Conclusions

The retroperitoneal laparoscopic approach for nephrectomy in patients with ADPKD emerges as a safe and effective technique, offering several advantages in terms of reduced blood loss, shorter hospital stays, and preservation of the peritoneal cavity. Current literature supports its adoption in selected cases and in experienced hands, highlighting its potential to improve perioperative outcomes and patient quality of life when compared to the open or transperitoneal approaches.

Number of patients	18
Indication for surgery	Pre-transplant space creation (13 cases); flank pain (3 cases); hematuria (2 cases)
Dialysis status	16 patients on dialysis: Hemodialysis (13) peritoneal dialysis (3)
Charlson Comorbidity Index	Median score: 4 (range: 4–5)
Mean hemoglobin (Hb)	11.3 g/dL ± 1.4
Mean renal volume (CT scan)	2,870 cc (range: 1,080–5,400)
Conversion to open surgery	Not required
Intraoperative complications	None
Mean operative time	149 minutes (range: 116–174 minutes)
Mean cyst suction volume	1,290 cc (range: 500–2,500 cc)
Mean final renal volume	810 cc (range: 477–1,164 cc)
Mean length of incision	7.3 cm (range: 7–8 cm)
Median first passage of flatus	Post-operative day (POD) 1 (all cases).
Median first passage of stool	POD 3 (range: 2–4)
Mean highest VAS score	POD 1: 2.8 (range: 1–5); POD 2: 2.8 (range: 2–5); POD 3: 2.3 (range: 1–5)
Mean Hb drop	2.5 g/dL
Complications	Two patients had more than two complications (Clavien-Dindo classification) – arteriovenous fistula
Transfusions	Four patients received one unit of red blood cells
Infective complications	None
Median length of hospital stay	Six days (range: 3–9 days)
Complications within 30 days	None

Table 2.
Patient characteristics.

Author details

Giovanni Busacca[1*], Ivano Morra[1], Luciano Ola[1], Bianca Sabrina Ribolzi[2] and Ettore Dalmasso[1]

1 Santa Croce e Carle Hospital, Department of Surgery, Division of Urology, Cuneo, Italy

2 Department of Urology, San Luigi Gonzaga Hospital, University of Turin, Orbassano, Italy

*Address all correspondence to: giovanni.busacca95@gmail.com

References

[1] Torres VE, Ahn C, Barten TRM, Brosnahan G, Cadnapaphornchai MA, Chapman AB, Cornec-Le Gall E, Drenth JPH, Gansevoort RT, Harris PC, Harris T, Horie S, Liebau MC, Liew M, Mallett AJ, Mei C, Mekahli D, Odland D, Ong ACM. KDIGO 2025 clinical practice guideline for the evaluation, management, and treatment of autosomal dominant polycystic kidney disease (ADPKD): Executive summary. Vicente E Torres 1, Curie Ahn 2, Thijs R M Barten 3, Godela Brosnahan 4, Melissa A Cadnapaphornchai 5, Arlene B Chapman 6. Kidney International. 2025;**107**(2):234–254. DOI: 10.1016/j.kint.2024.07.010

[2] Torres VE, Harris PC. Autosomal dominant polycystic kidney disease: The last 3 years. Kidney International. 2009;**76**(2):149–168. DOI: 10.1038/ki.2009.128

[3] Ryu SJ. Intracranial hemorrhage in patients with polycystic kidney disease. Stroke. 1990;**21**(2):291–294. DOI: 10.1161/01.str.21.2.291

[4] Harris Peter C, Torres VE, Adam MP, Feldman J, Mirzaa GM. Polycystic Kidney Disease, Autosomal Dominant. In: Adam MP, Bick S, Mirzaa GM. GeneReviews®. Seattle: University of Washington, Seattle; 1993

[5] Wisenbaugh ES, Tyson MD, Castle EP, Humphreys MR, Andrews PE. Massive renal size is not a contraindication to a laparoscopic approach for bilateral native nephrectomies in autosomal dominant polycystic kidney disease (ADPKD). BJU International. 2015;**115**(5):796–801. DOI: 10.1111/bju.12821

[6] Guo P, Xu W, Li H, Ni S, Ren M. Laparoscopic nephrectomy versus open nephrectomy for patients with autosomal dominant polycystic kidney disease: A systematic review and meta-analysis. PLoS One. 2015;**10**(6): e0129317. DOI: 10.1371/journal.pone.0129317

[7] Bennett AH, Stewart W, Lazarus JM. Bilateral nephrectomy in patients with polycystic renal disease. Surgery, Gynecology & Obstetrics. 1973;**137**(5):819–820

[8] Kikkawa K, Yamamoto H, Kohjimoto Y, Hara I. Laparoscopic nephrectomy via the retroperitoneal approach for autosomal dominant polycystic kidney disease after renal transplant: A case report. Experimental and Clinical Transplantation: Official Journal of the Middle East Society for Organ Transplantation. 2024;**22**(2):156–159. DOI: 10.6002/ect.2024.0020

[9] Wyler SF, Bachmann A, Ruszat R, Forster T, Hudolin T, Gasser TC, Sulser T. Retroperitoneoscopic nephrectomy for autosomal dominant polycystic kidney disease: Initial experience. Urologia Internationalis. 2007;**79**(2):137–141. DOI: 10.1159/000106327

[10] Gamé X, Vaessen C, Mouzin M, Mallet R, Malavaud B, Sarramon J-P, Rischmann P. Retroperitoneal laparoscopic nephrectomy fo polycystic kidney: Preliminary results. Progres En Urologie : Journal de l'Association Francaise D'urologie Et de la Societe Francaise D'urologie. 2003;**13**(2): 215–221

[11] Lyu J, Du C-K, Zhu Y. Comparison between retroperitoneal laparoscopic nephrectomy and traditional open nephrectomy to treat polycystic kidney disease before kidney transplantation. Urology Journal. 2024;**21**(2):74–79. DOI: 10.22037/uj.v20i.7826

[12] Chen K, Tan YG, Tan D, Pek G, Huang HH, Sim SPA. Predictors and outcomes of laparoscopic nephrectomy in autosomal dominant polycystic kidney disease. Investigative and Clinical Urology. 2018;**59**(4):238–245. DOI: 10.4111/icu.2018.59.4.238

[13] Abraham GP, Siddaiah AT, Das K, Ramaswami K, George DP, Thampan O. Laparoscopic nephrectomy for autosomal dominant polycystic kidneys in patients with end-stage renal disease on maintenance hemodialysis: 10-year single surgeon experience from an Indian center. Journal of Minimal Access Surgery. 2015;**11**(3):187–192. DOI: 10.4103/0972-9941.140217

[14] Benoit T, Peyronnet B, Roumiguie M, et al. Laparoscopic nephrectomy for polycystic kidney: Comparison of the transperitoneal and retroperitoneal approaches. World Journal of Urology. 2016;**34**(7): 901–906. DOI: 10.4103/0972-9941. 140217

[15] Bansal RK, Kapoor A. Laparoscopic nephrectomy for massive polycystic kidney disease: Updated technique and outcomes. Canadian Urological Association Journal. 2014;**8**(9-10): 341–345. DOI: 10.5489/cuaj.2097

[16] Lee DS, Kim HY, Lee S-J. Retroperitoneoscopic nephrectomy for huge autosomal-dominant polycystic kidney disease using morcellator. International Brazilian Journal of Urology. 2018;**44**(3): 651–652. DOI: 10.1590/S1677-5538. IBJU.2017.0258

[17] Cooksey R, Woodward MN. Laparoscopic-assisted retroperitoneal nephrectomy in autosomal recessive polycystic kidney disease. Journal of Pediatric Urology. 2015;**11**(6):366–367. DOI: 10.1016/j.jpurol.2015.08.009

[18] Hemal AK, Gupta NP, Rajeev TP, Aron M, Bhowmik D, Jain R. Retroperitoneoscopic Managementof InfectedCysts in Adult Polycystic Kidney Disease. Urologia Internationalis. 1999;**62**(1):40–43. DOI: 10.1159/000030354

Chapter 3

Current Surgical Treatment of Endometrial Carcinoma: The Role of Robotic Surgery

Elias Tsakos, Emmanouil Xydias, Dimitrios Balafoutas, Nikolaos Vlahos and Ralf Joukhadar

Abstract

Endometrial cancer is among the most common malignancies in women, and its incidence is on the rise. Treatment is primarily surgical, with hysterectomy, sentinel lymph node biopsy, and lymphadenectomy performed either by laparotomy or laparoscopy. Robotic surgery constitutes a novel approach to endometrial cancer treatment, promising to combine the efficacy of open surgery with the swift recovery and lower morbidity of minimally invasive techniques. Literature data suggest that robotic surgery is associated with better surgical outcomes, including reduced blood loss, lower complication rates, decreased transfusion rates, shorter length of hospital stay, and lower re-admission rates compared to open surgery. This is also the case for laparoscopy with regard to the length of hospital stay and the rate of conversion to open surgery. The surgical benefits of robotic surgery seem even more pronounced for obese and elderly endometrial cancer patients. Robotic surgery also offers improved pain-related outcomes, with significantly lower opioid consumption and reduced pain intensity compared to both alternatives. Oncological outcomes appear consistent regardless of the surgical approach, with the exception of a benefit in overall survival and recurrence rates for robotic surgery compared to laparotomy. Minimally invasive surgery appears to be the way forward in the treatment of endometrial cancer, with robotic surgery in particular offering several advantages over conventional alternatives, especially for high-risk patient subgroups. Additional studies accounting for disease surgical and molecular classification stages will assist in further investigating the benefits of modern technology and in establishing additional patient subcategories who would benefit most from the application of robotic technology.

Keywords: endometrial cancer, robotic surgery, surgical complications, overall survival, laparoscopy, laparotomy

1. Introduction

Endometrial cancer constitutes the sixth most common malignancy in females, with an estimated incidence of 8.7 cases per 100,000 women (age-standardized rate)

[1]. It is estimated that every woman has a cumulative lifetime risk of 3% of being diagnosed with endometrial cancer, with the average age of diagnosis being 61 years [2]. Endometrial cancer incidence is on the rise, with obesity, hormone replacement therapy, and advanced age constituting risk factors for its manifestation [3]. Prognosis largely depends on early diagnosis, as locally contained disease has significantly higher relative survival rates compared to regional and distant metastases [4] and effective surgical treatment [2].

Several advances in medical technology have allowed for improved prognosis of endometrial cancer in recent years, via breakthroughs in both its diagnosis and treatment. With regard to diagnosis, the advent of three-dimensional ultrasound, a modality with several applications in benign gynecology [5, 6], has shown promise in endometrial cancer diagnosis and classification [7, 8]. Most notably, however, this is true for endometrial cancer surgical treatment via the use of robotic surgical systems, the newest advancement in the field of Minimally Invasive Gynecology, with several technical advantages over more traditional techniques [9]. In this chapter, we shall analyze the role that robotic surgery can play in the treatment of endometrial cancer.

2. Surgical treatment of endometrial cancer: The status quo

The primary therapeutic modality employed in the treatment of endometrial cancer is surgical intervention, most commonly total hysterectomy, with non-interventional techniques such as chemotherapy, radiotherapy, and brachytherapy being utilized in the context of adjuvant or neo-adjuvant treatment [2]. This approach ensures complete resection of the primary tumor site and is supplemented by additional resection of surrounding lymphovascular tissue (lymphadenectomy) in the pelvis and para-aortically in order to ensure improved local control [2]. Since extensive lymphadenectomy is associated with increased operative time and patient morbidity, sentinel lymph node biopsy constitutes the modern standard of endometrial cancer staging, facilitating the assessment of lymphovascular expansion of the primary tumor with a high negative predictive value (approaching 99%), thus reducing the rate of needless lymphadenectomies [10].

Traditionally, total hysterectomy with or without lymphadenectomy for endometrial cancer is performed via laparotomy (open surgery), as direct access to the peritoneal cavity facilitates complex surgical maneuvers and ensures satisfactory oncological outcomes. However, the open approach has been associated with increased patient morbidity and longer hospital stays [11], highlighting the need for less invasive alternatives. This need has been met over the years by advances made in the field of minimally invasive surgery, and in particular, laparoscopy. This approach constitutes an alternative surgical option, with reduced surgical injury, swifter recovery times, and superior esthetic results [11]. However, laparoscopy does come with certain limitations regarding its oncological efficacy, limiting its recommended application to early-stage disease, according to European Guidelines [12], where it has proven to be safe and effective [13, 14]. In recent years, the development of robotic surgery holds the promise of combining the surgical efficacy and control of open surgery with the safety and recovery time of minimally invasive approaches.

3. Robotics in the modern gynecological surgery landscape

Robotic surgery was first made widely available during the 2000s with the advent of the da Vinci® Surgical System by Intuitive Surgical [15], and since then its application has expanded to multiple different surgical specialties, including general surgery, urological surgery, cardiothoracic surgery, head and neck surgery, and finally gynecological surgery [9].

A robotic surgical system includes several components for the purpose of improved control and surgeon ergonomics:

- Robotic arms: They carry the endoscopic surgical instruments and camera used for all surgical maneuvers. With the newer systems, all instruments and the camera are interchangeable between the four arms, facilitating several different arrangements for various interventions [9]. The robotic arms need to be docked onto specialized laparoscopic ports prior to the start of the procedure (**Figure 1**).

- Surgical instruments: Including most conventional endoscopic surgical instruments (forceps, needle driver, scissors, etc.), with the added benefit of articulation mimicking wrist movements compared to the rigid, non-articulating instruments of conventional laparoscopy [9].

- Surgical console: The center of the robotic surgical system, the console facilitates control of the robotic arms and instruments via specialized ergonomic hand controls and foot pedals. This arrangement also facilitates control of the endoscopic camera in addition to the three surgical instruments, contrary to conventional laparoscopy, where a second surgeon is required (**Figure 1**) [16].

- Endoscopic camera: Three-dimensional, high-resolution imaging of the surgical site facilitates improved depth perception and magnification, thus allowing safe and complex surgical maneuvers [9, 16].

- Integrated near-infrared imaging capabilities, allowing for the detection of infused indocyanine green (ICG), a modality with several applications, particularly in endometrial cancer surgery (**Figure 2**).

These components confer a plethora of technical and practical advantages with regard to operative efficiency, safety, and comfort. Namely, the most important is the accuracy of surgical movements, thanks to the master controls and integrated tremor filters, which translate the natural, intuitive hand movements into robotic arm movements without tremor, thus offering stability and reducing surgical trauma [16]. The improved surgical control is further enhanced via the three-dimensional vision integrated into the system, improving spatial awareness and further limiting healthy tissue injury [17]. Finally, the ergonomic controls and seated position of the surgeon reduce fatigue and permit lengthy operation times, which are particularly relevant for challenging surgeries and high-volume centers [9]. These advantages hold the potential to significantly improve surgical outcomes for endometrial cancer treatment, with a reduction in morbidity, complications, and re-admission rates, while maintaining an acceptable cost-effectiveness ratio [18].

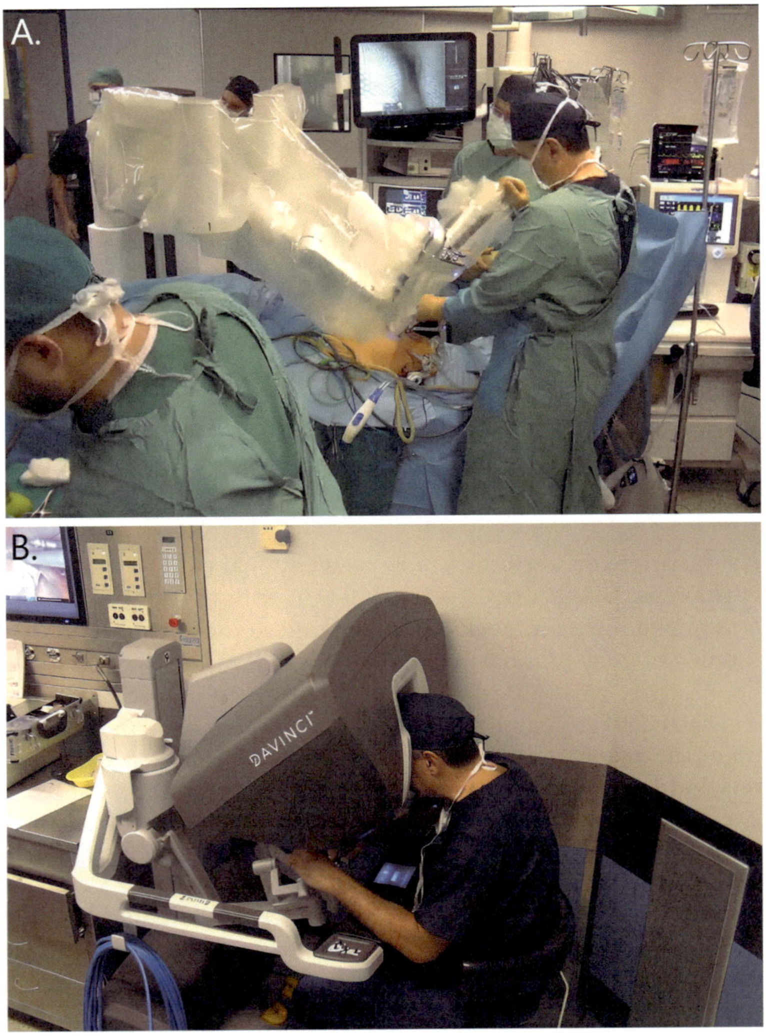

Figure 1.
Operating room images of the da Vinci X® robotic surgical system: (A) patient cart positioning and surgical arms docking, (B) surgical console providing control of all four arms and three-dimensional vision of the surgical field.

4. Efficacy of robotic hysterectomy in the treatment of endometrial cancer

4.1 Literature review

A systematic literature review and meta-analysis were performed to collect and analyze all available evidence on the safety and efficacy of robotic surgery in the treatment of endometrial cancer. Studies that included adult women diagnosed with endometrial cancer, treated with robotic surgery, and compared to another group

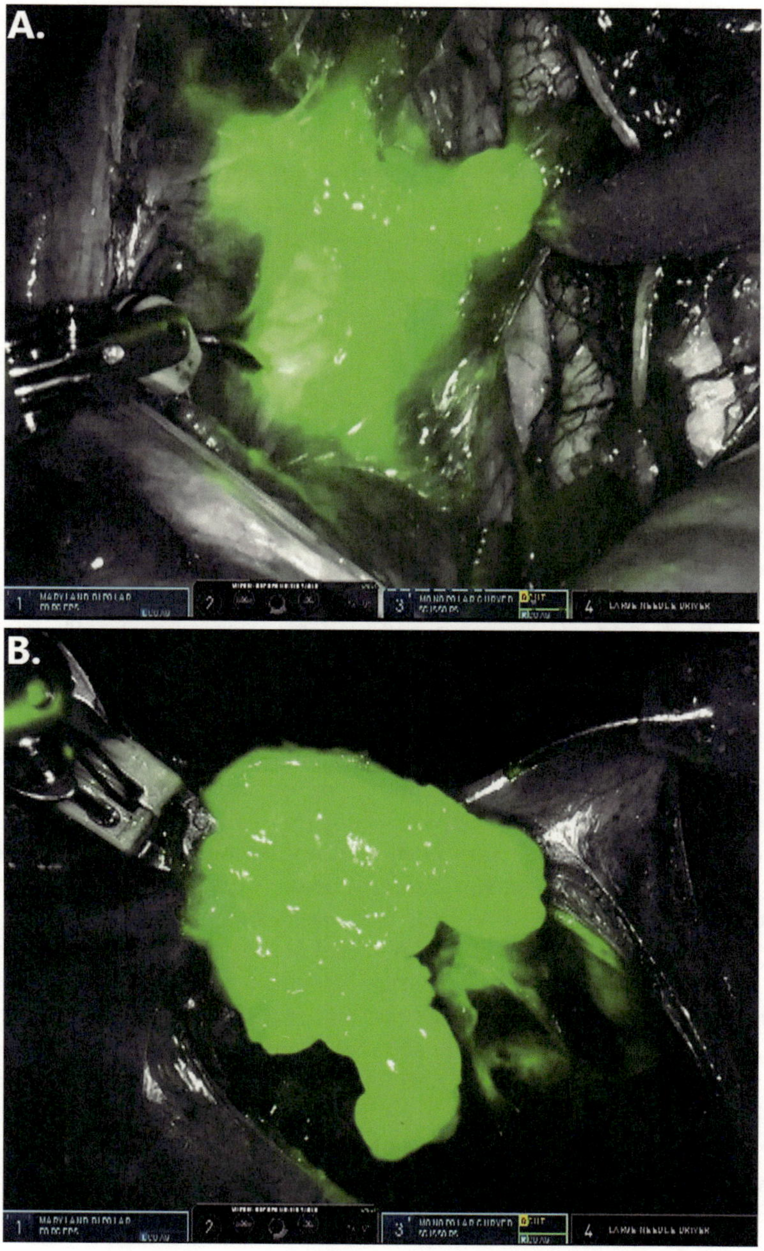

Figure 2.
Application of indocyanine green infusion and near-infrared imaging facilitated by the Firefly® system of the da Vinci® surgical platform for: (A) the identification and (B) the excision of marked sentinel lymph nodes.

treated with either laparoscopy or laparotomy were eligible for inclusion. The primary outcomes of interest for this review were:

Surgical parameters (blood loss, operative time, complications, readmission, etc.), pain-related parameters (opioid consumption, reported pain, etc.) and oncological.

Parameters (survival, recurrence, etc.) were evaluated. Relevant studies were searched for in MEDLINE/PubMed, Ovid, Web of Science, CINAHL, and Scopus with the use of the following search algorithm: (Robotic odds ratio [OR], robotic-assisted OR, robotically-assisted OR, "robotic assisted" OR, "robotically assisted") AND (hysterectomy OR surgery) AND (endometri* OR uter*) AND (cancer OR carcinoma OR malignancy OR neoplasia) AND (laparoscopic OR laparoscopy OR laparotomy OR open). The studies were assessed and meta-analyzed using random-effects meta-analysis. Weighted Mean Difference (WMD) and OR were the effect measures for the cumulative continuous and categorical outcomes, respectively.

From an initial pool of 4,412 studies, following systematic evaluation in accordance with the PRISMA 2020 Guidelines, ultimately, data from 82 studies were included in the review [19–111]. A detailed flowchart depicting the study evaluation and exclusion process, along with reasons for exclusion, is available in Appendix A. The eligible studies were performed between 2000 and 2018 and published from 2008 onward. In total, they included 146,128 women with endometrial cancer who underwent surgical treatment, 71,100 of whom underwent robotic, 26,815 laparoscopic, and 48,213 open surgery. The vast majority of studies utilized da Vinci Surgical Systems (several models, including standard, S, Si, X, and Xi). Number and placement of robotic ports varied amongst the studies, however most utilized 4–5 in total (3–4 robotic ports and one accessory port), placed most frequently on a straight line or arch, with the cameral port located at the level of the umbilicus or 1–2 cm above it, two robotic ports on either side, approximately 7–10 cm from the umbilicus port (mid-lateral position) and accessory port 5–7 cm from the robotic ones laterally on the abdominal wall. A fourth robotic port was placed by some investigators on the opposite side of the abdominal wall to the accessory port. Trocars for robotic instruments were 8 mm in diameter, camera port was 8 mm in newer models and 12 mm in older models (standard, S), and the accessory port was usually 12 mm. Regarding preferred robotic instruments, these also varied among the studies, however, the majority of surgeons utilized the following: Maryland bipolar forceps, fenestrated bipolar forceps (Cadiere), monopolar curved scissors, graspers, and needle driver. Where sufficient data were available, subanalysis of patients of advanced age (over 65 years) and obese patients (BMI >30) was performed, since advanced age and obesity are known risk factors for both endometrial cancer and increased surgical risk. This facilitated assessment of the performance of robotic surgery compared to the other two alternatives in a common and surgically challenging patient population.

4.2 Surgical outcomes

4.2.1 Meta-analysis results

Surgical outcomes represent the primary performance indices, on the basis of which assessment of different surgical techniques may take place. They are directly related to the immediate outcomes of surgery and are mostly associated with patient safety and recovery time.

Meta-analysis of the available literature data indicated that robotic hysterectomy (RH) had consistently longer operative times compared with both alternatives.

The difference in time was statistically significant but not clinically meaningful for the general endometrial cancer population (approximately 10 minutes longer). This trend was consistent in obese patients as well; however, RH lasted significantly longer compared to open hysterectomy (OH) (over 30 minutes on average). Regarding intra-operative blood loss, RH led to consistently less bleeding compared to both alternatives. This difference was statistically significant for both comparisons but was more clinically meaningful for RH versus OH (>130 ml) rather than laparoscopic hysterectomy (LH) (~15–40 ml). This trend was even more prominent in older and obese women, for whom RH caused over 200 ml less blood loss compared to OH. The need for transfusions was consistently less common for RH compared to OH by approximately 80%, regardless of the presence of advanced age or obesity; however, there were no differences versus LH.

Intra-operative complications showed no statistically significant differences among the different surgical methods and patient populations, with the exception of a ~35% reduction with RH compared to OH for the general population. Post-operative complications were consistently less common for RH compared to OH by approximately 70%; however, there were no differences when compared to LH. These observations were consistent across all patient subgroups. RH was ~60% less likely to lead to conversion to open surgery compared to LH for the general population. This was even more pronounced for obese patients, with 80% lower conversion rates.

With regard to hospitalization duration, RH was associated with an over 35-times higher same-day release rate compared to LH. Regarding re-admission after surgery, RH had nearly a 50% lower risk compared to OH; however, it was no different on this parameter when compared to LH. The most consistent benefit of RH, compared with both alternatives, was the length of hospital stay. Compared to OH, RH had a shorter stay by over 2.5 days and by 0.5 days compared to LH – both statistically and clinically significant differences. This difference was even more prominent for women of advanced age, for whom RH offered over 3 days shorter length of stay compared to OH and over 1.5 days compared to LH. A similar trend was observed for obese women as well, with over 3.3 days shorter stays compared to OH and close to 0.5 days compared to LH. These findings are summarized in **Table 1**.

4.2.2 Interpretation of findings

The present analysis indicated statistically significant differences between RH and both OH and LH with regard to operative time; however, this difference was not clinically meaningful. A statistically and clinically significant difference in operative time was, however, observed in obese women for RH compared to OH (approximately 30 min), while a clinically non-meaningful difference was observed compared to LH. This is consistent with the known challenges of minimally invasive surgery for obese patients, requiring additional time compared to normal-weight ones [21], and is to be expected to some degree. These findings are more or less consistent with those of other analyses, with robotic surgery having longer operative times, which are not very meaningful clinically [22]. Furthermore, operative time is directly related to the experience of the surgeon and OR team [23]; therefore, robotic surgery, being significantly more recent compared to both alternatives and the majority of authors reporting their first experience with the method, are factors likely to contribute to the observed differences.

Outcomes	**General population**		**Women >65y**		**Obese women (BMI >30)**	
	RH vs. OH	**RH vs. LH**	**RH vs. OH**	**RH vs. LH**	**RH vs. OH**	**RH vs. LH**
Operative time (WMD)	***N* = 6,684, WMD = +12.83 min, *p* <0.001***	***N* = 9,987, WMD = +10.81 min, *p* <0.001***	N/A	N/A	***N* = 687, WMD = 34.03 min, *p* <0.001***	***N* = 1,505, WMD = 8.81 min, *p* <0.001***
Estimated Blood loss (WMD)	***N* = 5,380, WMD = -135.96 ml, *p* <0.001***	***N* = 7,829, WMD = -39.5 ml, *p* <0.001***	***N* = 533, WMD = -227.39 ml, *p* <0.001***	N/A	***N* = 687, WMD = -267.27 ml, *p* <0.001***	***N* = 1,554, WMD = -14.04 ml, *p* = 0.007***
Transfusion rate (OR)	***N* = 5,558, OR = 0.23, *p* <0.001***	*N* = 15,975, OR = 0.72, *p* = 0.066	***N* = 7,439, OR = 0.23, *p* <0.001***	*N* = 2021, OR = 0.82, *p* = 0.430	***N* = 530, OR = 0.18, *p* <0.001***	*N* = 761, OR = 3.50, *p* = 0.104
Intra-operative complications (OR)	***N* = 4,973, OR = 0.66, *p* = 0.036***	*N* = 20,550, OR = 0.80, *p* = 0.117	*N* = 7,535, OR = 1.14, *p* = 0.823	*N* = 2,166, OR = 0.82, *p* = 0.209	*N* = 473, OR = 1.12, *p* = 0.847	*N* = 1,319, OR = 1.04, *p* = 0.947
Post-operative complications (OR)	***N* = 11,135, OR = 0.32, *p* <0.001***	*N* = 13,589, OR = 0.85, *p* = 0.162	***N* = 7,717, OR = 0.30, *p* <0.001***	*N* = 2,209, OR = 1.10, *p* = 0.840	***N* = 687, OR = 0.30, *p* <0.001***	*N* = 1,328, OR = 0.67, *p* = 0.360
Conversion to open surgery (OR)	N/A	***N* = 18,437, OR = 0.41, *p* = 0.001***	N/A	N/A	N/A	***N* = 1,321, OR = 0.19, *p* <0.001***
Length of hospital stay (WMD)	***N* = 42,770, WMD = -2.55 days, *p* <0.001***	***N* = 43,105, WMD = -0.46 days, *p* <0.001***	***N* = 7717, WMD = -3.13 days, *p* <0.001***	***N* = 231, WMD = -1.76 days, *p* <0.001***	***N* = 637, WMD = -3.38 days, *p* <0.001***	***N* = 1,456, WMD = -0.46 days, *p* <0.001***
Same day release (OR)	N/A	**N = 1,205, OR = 37.68, *p* <0.001***	N/A	N/A	N/A	N/A
Re-admission (OR)	***N* = 40,734, OR = 0.51, *p* <0.001***	*N* = 35,652, OR = 1.00, *p* = 0.984	N/A	N/A	N/A	N/A

*RH: robotic hysterectomy, OH: open hysterectomy, LH: laparoscopic hysterectomy, WMD: weighted mean difference, OR: odds ratio, green: favors RH, red: does not favor RH, *: statistically significant difference, N: patient number for this comparison, N/A: not applicable or not available.*

Table 1.
Summary of meta-analysis results per comparison and per parameter for surgical outcomes.

With regard to intra-operative blood loss, the statistically significant advantage of RH was consistent with the findings of other meta-analyses on the topic [22], confirming the theory of less traumatic intervention facilitated via robotic surgery. However, the difference compared with LH may not be considered clinically meaningful, indicating that the primary advantage of less blood loss is conferred by the minimally invasive nature of the procedures alone and not the robotic system in particular. Similar findings regarding intra-operative bleeding have been observed in other robotic gynecological interventions as well, such as myomectomy, urogynecology, and other benign indications [24, 25]. This trend was even more pronounced for high surgical risk patients (>65 years and obese) compared to OH, indicating a significant advantage of RH for these patient categories in particular.

Intra-operative complication rates were significantly lower for RH compared to OH but were not different for LH. No differences were observed in either elderly patients or obese ones. These findings were consistent with the previously reported analysis by Liu et al. as far as OH was concerned; however, the investigators reported a statistically significant benefit of RH compared to LH as well (43% fewer intra-operative complications) [22], a discrepancy that could be attributed to newer studies included in the present analysis and methodological differences (separate analysis of high-risk patients). Transfusion and post-operative complication rate trends were more consistent with previously reported observations [22] and were significantly lower only when compared to OH. These results may indicate that, while minimally invasive techniques are associated with a significant, demonstrable decrease in complications [26], the particular technical features and benefits of the robotic system may not play as important a role as the minimal access nature of the surgery itself. A different trend was observed with regard to the conversion-to-open-surgery rate, an important complication associated with increased patient morbidity [27]. In particular, RH had significantly lower conversion rates compared with conventional LH, a trend consistent with the available literature [22], and was even more prominent for obese patients, with as much as an 80% reduced risk. Considering the fact that this sub-group of patients is already at increased surgical risk, a minimization of conversion rates and the associated morbidity [27] would be highly beneficial. This significant difference for obese patients in particular could be attributed to the particularly challenging entry process and establishment of pneumoperitoneum for this patient subgroup [28] and the potential role that the increased control and superior imaging capabilities of the robotic systems can play in this regard.

With regard to the final core surgical outcomes, the length of hospital stay was significantly shorter for RH compared to both OH and LH for all patient subgroups, a trend consistent with previous analyses [22]. This difference was more prominent in the comparison of RH and OH across all three subgroups. Furthermore, differences were even more pronounced for RH versus OH in elderly and obese patients, and for RH versus LH in elderly patients. All differences were clinically meaningful. The reduced length of stay for RH patients is an indirect indicator of reduced surgical morbidity and supports the proposed advantages of robotic surgery over conventional alternatives. This conclusion is further reinforced by the impressive 37-fold increase in the same-day discharge rate for RH compared to LH, although this should be interpreted with caution due to the smaller number of available studies and patients. Finally, the re-admission rate was significantly lower for RH compared with OH but was non-significant compared with LH. This is consistent with observations made by Liu et al. [22] and is an indicator of lower patient risk and lower costs as well, since total costs for patients with re-admission may be up to 60% higher compared to those without re-admission [29].

4.3 Pain-related outcomes

4.3.1 Meta-analysis results

Pain-related outcomes comprise a group of more indirect indices of surgical safety and efficacy, reflecting the extent of tissue trauma during surgery and the pain experienced by the patients. While they constitute more subjective outcomes compared to surgical ones, pain-related parameters are of great significance for patient experience and quality of life during the early post-operative period.

Therefore, they should not be ignored in the assessment of the efficacy of robotic surgery.

With regard to intra-operative use of opioids, a meta-analysis of two studies with 344 participants reported that patients who underwent RH required, on average, 2.02 fewer morphine milligram equivalents (MME) compared to those who underwent LH, although this was not a statistically significant difference. A similar trend was observed for RH versus OH, with data from a single study indicating that RH required 0.55 MME fewer compared to OH, although this was also non-significant ($p = 0.624$) [30]. However, post-operative consumption of opioids during PACU stay was significantly lower in RH patients compared to OH by 5.39 MME ($p < 0.001$) based on data from a single study [30]. This trend was consistent but less pronounced for the comparison of RH and LH, with 1.22 MME ($p = 0.029$), based on a meta-analysis of two studies [31, 32]. Finally, opioid consumption during post-operative stay at the surgical ward was significantly lower for RH compared to OH, with 19.4 MME lower consumption [30], and lower compared to LH by 0.33 MME [32], which was not statistically significant.

With regard to subjective pain assessment after surgery, RH was associated with less pain by 0.33 units on a 10-point scale, which was a statistically significant difference ($p = 0.038$) [33]. This trend was similar for the comparison with LH, with data from a meta-analysis of three studies and 819 patients indicating 0.63 points lower perceived pain intensity for RH patients ($p < 0.001$) [31, 32, 34]. Regarding perceived pain throughout the first 24 hours post-operatively, data from two studies and 386 patients indicated that RH patients reported lower pain scores by 0.55 points on a 10-point scale, which was statistically significant ($p < 0.001$) [33, 35]. This trend was consistent for the comparison with LH as well, with 0.51 points of difference, based on a meta-analysis of data from four studies and 539 patients [32, 35–37]. These results are summarized in **Table 2**.

4.3.2 Interpretation of findings

Significantly fewer data were available for this category of outcomes compared to surgical ones, indicating that results and conclusions from this category may require further investigation for definitive conclusions. Overall, all outcomes were more favorable for RH compared to both alternatives; however, they were statistically significant in specific cases. Notable examples include significantly lower doses of opioids during PACU stay for both comparisons and in the surgical ward for the OH comparison alone. Furthermore, post-operative pain scores were significantly lower for RH compared with either alternative.

Outcomes	RH vs. OH	RH vs. LH
Intra-op opioids (WMD)	N = 133 (single study), WMD = -0.55 MME, p = 0.624	N = 344, WMD = -2.02 MME, p = 0.283
PACU opioids (WMD)	**N = 133 (single study), WMD = -5.39 MME, p <0.001***	**N = 344, WMD = -1.22 MME, p = 0.023***
Recovery opioids (WMD)	**N = 133 (single study), WMD = -19.4 MME, p <0.001***	N = 297 (single study), WMD = 0.33 MME, p = 0.729
Post-op VAS (WMD)	**N = 365 (single study) WMD = - 0.3, p = 0.038***	**N = 819, WMD = -0.63, p <0.001***
First 24 h VAS (WMD)	**N = 386, WMD = -0.55, p <0.001***	**N = 539, WMD = -0.51, P = 0.002***

*RH: robotic hysterectomy, OH: open hysterectomy, LH: laparoscopic hysterectomy, WMD: weighted mean difference, OR: odds ratio, green: favors RH, red: does not favor RH, *: statistically significant difference, N: patient number for this comparison.*

Table 2.
Summary of meta-analysis results per comparison and per parameter for pain-related outcomes.

These outcomes likely reflect the reduced healthy tissue trauma achieved via robotic surgery, through improved control of movement and better visualization of the surgical field [9]. With regard to OH, the utilization of small incisions and the limited exposure of the peritoneal cavity to the outside contribute to the reduction of surgical stress and thus post-operative pain and need for analgesia [38].

4.4 Oncological outcomes

4.4.1 Meta-analysis results

Oncological outcomes constitute the most important measures of success following endometrial cancer treatment. While they are multifactorial outcomes, affected by several different parameters, including adjuvant treatment and disease stage, they also reflect surgical efficacy and are important when selecting a surgical route.

With regard to recurrence rates, RH was associated with significantly lower odds compared to OH, with OR: 0.62 (p <0.001). While this trend was maintained for the comparison with LH, it was not statistically significant (OR: 0.87, p = 0.169). With regard to survival statistics, 5 year estimates were utilized. In order to ensure that no other confounding factors affected the results, a meta-analysis of the reported hazard ratios (HR) of the individual studies was performed, utilizing estimates from multivariate analyses that accounted for all confounders. For 5 year disease-free survival, no statistically significant differences were observed for RH compared to either OH or LH, with a non-significant trend favoring robotics (HR: 0.78, p = 0.214 and HR: 0.81, p = 0.166, respectively). Finally, with regard to 5-year overall survival, RH was superior to OH with HR: 0.85 (p <0.001); however, it had no significant differences compared to LH (HR: 0.92, p = 0.528). These results are summarized in **Table 3**.

Outcomes	RH vs. OH	RH vs. LH
Recurrence rate (OR)	**N = 3,466, OR = 0.68, p <0.001***	N = 6,192, OR = 0.87, p = 0.169
5-year disease free survival (HR)	N = 700, HR = 0.78, p = 0.214	N = 2,785, HR = 0.81, p = 0.166
5-year overall survival (OR)	**N = 96,163, HR = 0.85, p <0.001***	N = 5,517, HR = 0.92, p = 0.528

*RH: robotic hysterectomy, OH: open hysterectomy, LH: laparoscopic hysterectomy, OR: odds ratio, HR: hazard ratio, green: favors RH, red: does not favor RH, *: statistically significant difference, N: patient number for this comparison.*

Table 3.
Summary of meta-analysis results per comparison and per parameter for oncological outcomes.

4.4.2 Interpretation of findings

Oncological outcomes indicated an overall favorable trend toward robotic surgery, which, however, was not statistically significant for the majority of comparisons. Exceptions to that were the recurrence rate and overall survival of RH compared to OH, which were significantly better. These findings are consistent with the meta-analysis by Fu et al. [39], who argue that the apparent benefit of RH compared to OH could be attributed to factors such as improved surgical outcomes and safety, a larger number of collected lymph nodes, a higher likelihood of timely adjuvant treatment (due to faster recovery from surgery), higher socioeconomic status associated with better access to treatment, and greater confidence with a positive attitude associated with patients undergoing RH [39].

5. Conclusions

Endometrial cancer is a common malignancy with increasing incidence and is associated with common risk factors such as advanced age and obesity. Its treatment is primarily surgical and is complicated by the fact that its common risk factors also constitute factors associated with increased surgical risk. Therefore, a safe and effective treatment modality is paramount in ensuring optimal outcomes. This modality could be robotic surgery, the latest advancement in minimally invasive gynecological surgery. The present review indicated that RH outperformed OH on almost all surgical, pain-related, and even oncological outcomes, thus confirming its value over the more invasive conventional alternative. The performance of RH may have been comparable to that of LH; however, the reduced blood loss, conversion to open surgery, and length of hospital stay, particularly for high-risk patient subgroups, are indicative of the value of the application of robotics in this field. Additional studies should aim to further elucidate this application of modern technology, particularly with regard to high-risk patient subgroups.

Appendix

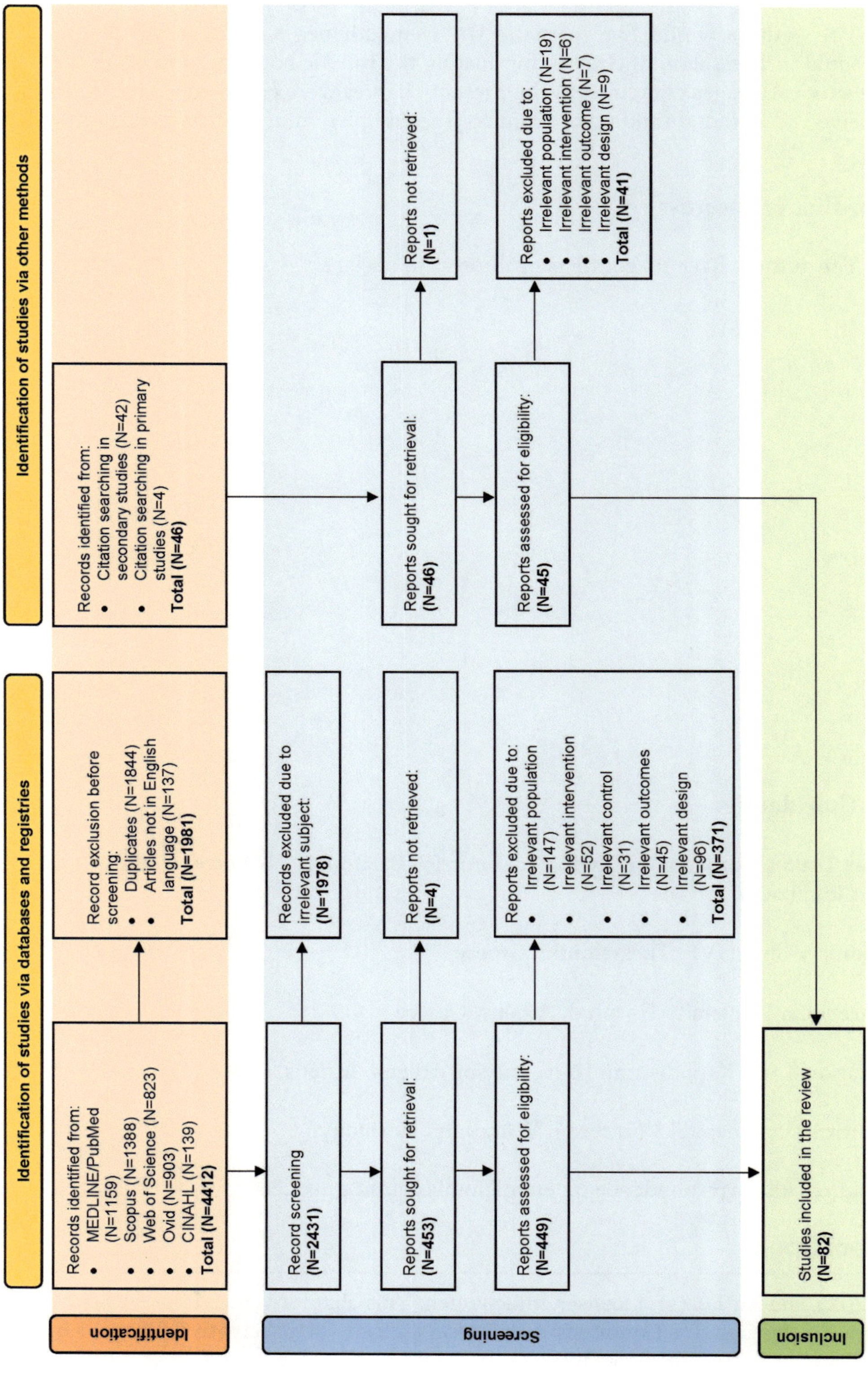

Appendix A.
PRISMA 2020 flowchart demonstrating the study evaluation, inclusion, and exclusion process for the present systematic review.

Acknowledgments

The authors would like to thank Dr. Demosthenes Katsarkas and St. Luke's Hospital in Thessaloniki, Greece, for hosting the robotic equipment through which the surgical images contained in the present chapter were collected. The authors received no external funding or grant for the completion of this chapter.

Conflict of interest

The authors have no conflicts of interest to declare.

Author details

Elias Tsakos[1], Emmanouil Xydias[1*], Dimitrios Balafoutas[2], Nikolaos Vlahos[3], and Ralf Joukhadar[4]

1 EmbryoClinic IVF, Thessaloniki, Greece

2 Aretaieio University Hospital, Athens, Greece

3 National and Kapodistrian University of Athens, Athens, Greece

4 University Hospital Würzburg, Würzburg, Germany

*Address all correspondence to: emmanouilxydias@gmail.com

References

[1] Sung H, Ferlay J, Siegel RL, Laversanne M, Soerjomataram I, Jemal A, et al. Global cancer statistics 2020: GLOBOCAN estimates of incidence and mortality worldwide for 36 cancers in 185 countries. Ca A Cancer Journal for Clinicians. 2021;**71**(3): 209–249. DOI: 10.3322/caac.21660

[2] Crosbie EJ, Kitson SJ, McAlpine JN, Mukhopadhyay A, Powell ME, Singh N. Endometrial cancer. The Lancet. 2022;**399**(10333):1412–1428. DOI: 10.1016/s0140-6736(22)00323-3

[3] Doll A, Abal M, Rigau M, Monge M, Gonzalez M, Demajo S, et al. Novel molecular profiles of endometrial cancer —new light through old windows. The Journal of Steroid Biochemistry and Molecular Biology. 2008;**108**(3-5):221–229. DOI: 10.1016/j.jsbmb.2007.09.020

[4] Surveillance Research Program NCI. SEER*Explorer: An interactive website for SEER cancer statistics 2023 [updated 2023 November 16]. Data source(s): SEER Incidence Data, 2022 Submission (1975-2020), SEER 22 registries (excluding Illinois and Massachusetts). Expected Survival Life Tables by Socio-Economic Standards. Available from: https://seer.cancer.gov/statistics-network/explorer/

[5] Xydias EM, Liasidi P-N, Papageorgouli D, Tsakos E, Gouliopoulos N, Thanasas I, et al. Three-dimensional transvaginal ultrasound versus MRI in the diagnosis and classification of congenital uterine anomalies: A systematic review and meta-analysis. European Journal of Obstetrics & Gynecology and Reproductive Biology. 2025;**312**:114560. DOI: 10.1016/j.ejogrb.2025.114560

[6] Ziogas A, Xydias E, Tsakos E. Novel Methods in the Diagnosis of PCOS: The Role of 3D Ultrasonographic Modalities. In: Wang Z, editor. Polycystic Ovary Syndrome - Functional Investigation and Clinical Application. Rijeka: IntechOpen. 2022;4–8

[7] Xydias EM, Kalantzi S, Tsakos E, Ntanika A, Beis N, Prior M, et al. Comparison of 3D ultrasound, 2D ultrasound and 3D Doppler in the diagnosis of endometrial carcinoma in patients with uterine bleeding: A systematic review and meta-analysis. European Journal of Obstetrics & Gynecology and Reproductive Biology. 2022;**277**:42–52

[8] Ziogas A, Xydias E, Kalantzi S, Papageorgouli D, Liasidi PN, Lamari I, et al. The diagnostic accuracy of 3D ultrasound compared to 2D ultrasound and MRI in the assessment of deep myometrial invasion in endometrial cancer patients: A systematic review. Taiwanese Journal of Obstetrics and Gynecology. 2022;**61**(5):746–754. DOI: 10.1016/j.tjog.2022.06.002

[9] Reddy K, Gharde P, Tayade H, Patil M, Reddy LS, Surya D. Advancements in robotic surgery: A comprehensive overview of current utilizations and upcoming frontiers. Cureus. 2023; **15**(12):e50415. DOI: 10.7759/cureus.50415

[10] Leitao Jr MM, Khoury-Collado F, Gardner G, Sonoda Y, Brown CL, Alektiar KM, et al. Impact of incorporating an algorithm that utilizes sentinel lymph node mapping during minimally invasive procedures on the detection of stage IIIC endometrial cancer. Gynecologic Oncology.

2013;**129**(1):38–41. DOI: 10.1016/j.ygyno.2013.01.002

[11] de la Orden SG, Reza MM, Blasco JA, Andradas E, Callejo D, Pérez T. Laparoscopic hysterectomy in the treatment of endometrial cancer: A systematic review. Journal of Minimally Invasive Gynecology. 2008;**15**(4):395–401. DOI: 10.1016/j.jmig.2008.04.018

[12] Concin N, Creutzberg CL, Vergote I, Cibula D, Mirza MR, Marnitz S, et al. ESGO/ESTRO/ESP guidelines for the management of patients with endometrial carcinoma. Virchows Archiv : an International Journal of Pathology. 2021;**478**(2):153–190. DOI: 10.1007/s00428-020-03007-z

[13] Togami S, Kawamura T, Fukuda M, Yanazume S, Kamio M, Kobayashi H. Learning curve and surgical outcomes for laparoscopic surgery, including pelvic lymphadenectomy, for early stage endometrial cancer. Japanese Journal of Clinical Oncology. 2019;**49**(6):521–524. DOI: 10.1093/jjco/hyz027

[14] Walker JL, Piedmonte MR, Spirtos NM, Eisenkop SM, Schlaerth JB, Mannel RS, et al. Recurrence and survival after random assignment to laparoscopy versus laparotomy for comprehensive surgical staging of uterine cancer: Gynecologic oncology group LAP2 study. Journal of Clinical Oncology. 2012;**30**(7):695–700. DOI: 10.1200/jco.2011.38.8645

[15] George EI, Brand TC, LaPorta A, Marescaux J, Satava RM. Origins of robotic surgery: From skepticism to standard of care. Journal of the Society of Laparoendoscopic Surgeons. 2018;**22**(4). DOI: 10.4293/jsls.2018.00039

[16] Morris B. Robotic surgery: Applications, limitations, and impact on surgical education. Medscape General Medicine. 2005;7(3):72

[17] Bhayani SB, Andriole GL. Three-dimensional (3D) vision: Does it improve laparoscopic skills? An assessment of a 3d head-mounted visualization system. Reviews in Urology. 2005;7(4):211–214

[18] Casarin J, Song C, Multinu F, Cappuccio S, Liu E, Butler KA, et al. Implementing robotic surgery for uterine cancer in the United States: Better outcomes without increased costs. Gynecologic Oncology. 2020;**156**(2):451–458. DOI: 10.1016/j.ygyno.2019.11.016

[19] Abel MK, Chan JK, Chow S, Darcy K, Tian C, Kapp DS, et al. Trends and survival outcomes of robotic, laparoscopic, and open surgery for stage II uterine cancer. International Journal of Gynecological Cancer. 2020;**30**(9):1347–1355. DOI: 10.1136/ijgc-2020-001646

[20] Zakhari A, Czuzoj-Shulman N, Spence AR, Gotlieb WH, Abenhaim HA. Laparoscopic and robot-assisted hysterectomy for uterine cancer: A comparison of costs and complications. American Journal of Obstetrics and Gynecology. 2015;**213**(5):665.e1–7. DOI: 10.1016/j.ajog.2015.07.004

[21] Khoiwal K, Kapoor N, Gaurav A, R K, Reddy KK, Chaturvedi J. The effect of body mass index on peri-operative parameters of total laparoscopic hysterectomy: An institutional experience. Cureus. 2021; **13**(6):e15558. DOI: 10.7759/cureus.15558

[22] Liu H, Cao Y, Li L, Bai Y, Liu J. Effectiveness of robotic surgery for

endometrial cancer: A systematic review and meta-analysis. Archives of Gynecology & Obstetrics. 2022;**305**(4):837–850. DOI: 10.1007/s00404-021-06229-x

[23] Panico G, Mastrovito S, Campagna G, Monterossi G, Costantini B, Gioè A, et al. Robotic docking time with the Hugo™ RAS system in gynecologic surgery: A procedure independent learning curve using the cumulative summation analysis (CUSUM). Journal of Robotic Surgery. 2023;**17**(5):2547–2554. DOI: 10.1007/s11701-023-01693-w

[24] Tsakos E, Xydias EM, Ziogas AC, Bimpa K, Doumouchtsis SK, Karydas G, et al. Surgical and quality of life outcomes following robotic-assisted (da Vinci) laparoscopic repair of vesicovaginal fistula: A case report and video demonstration. Cureus. 2023;**15**(7):e42171. DOI: 10.7759/cureus.42171

[25] Tsakos E, Xydias EM, Ziogas AC, Sorrentino F, Nappi L, Vlachos N, et al. Multi-port robotic-assisted laparoscopic myomectomy: A systematic review and meta-analysis of comparative clinical and fertility outcomes. Journal of Clinical Medicine. 2023;**12**(12). DOI: 10.3390/jcm12124134

[26] Kelly EC, Winick-Ng J, McClure JA, Peart T, Chou Q, MacMillan B, et al. Hysterectomy in ontario: A population-based study of outcomes and complications in minimally invasive compared with abdominal approaches. Journal of Obstetrics and Gynaecology Canada. 2019;**41**(8):1168–1176. DOI: 10.1016/j.jogc.2018.10.026

[27] Lim CS, Mowers EL, Mahnert N, Skinner BD, Kamdar N, Morgan DM, et al. Risk factors and outcomes for conversion to laparotomy of laparoscopic hysterectomy in benign gynecology. Obstetrics & Gynecology. 2016;**128**(6):1295–1305. DOI: 10.1097/aog.0000000000001743

[28] McIlwaine K, Cameron M, Readman E, Manwaring J, Maher P. The effect of patient body mass index on surgical difficulty in gynaecological laparoscopy. Gynecological Surgery. 2011;**8**(2):145–149. DOI: 10.1007/s10397-010-0636-6

[29] Zheng S, Hanchate A, Shwartz M. One-year costs of medical admissions with and without a 30-day readmission and enhanced risk adjustment. BMC Health Services Research. 2019;**19**(1):155. DOI: 10.1186/s12913-019-3983-7

[30] Agarwal R, Rajanbabu A, Unnikrishnan UG. A retrospective evaluation of the perioperative drug use and comparison of its cost in robotic vs open surgery for endometrial cancer. Journal of Robotic Surgery. 2018;**12**(4):665–672. DOI: 10.1007/s11701-018-0799-0

[31] Fleming ND, Havrilesky LJ, Valea FA, Allen TK, Broadwater G, Bland A, et al. Analgesic and antiemetic needs following minimally invasive vs open staging for endometrial cancer. American Journal of Obstetrics and Gynecology. 2011;**204**(1):65.e1–6. DOI: 10.1016/j.ajog.2010.08.020

[32] Turner TB, Habib AS, Broadwater G, Valea FA, Fleming ND, Ehrisman JA, et al. Postoperative pain scores and narcotic use in robotic-assisted versus laparoscopic hysterectomy for endometrial cancer staging. Journal of Minimally Invasive Gynecology. 2015;**22**(6):1004–1010. DOI: 10.1016/j.jmig.2015.05.003

[33] Chiou HY, Chiu LH, Chen CH, Yen YK, Chang CW, Liu WM. Comparing robotic surgery with laparoscopy and laparotomy for endometrial cancer management: A cohort study. International Journal of Surgery. 2015;**13**:17–22. DOI: 10.1016/j.ijsu.2014.11.015

[34] Leitao Jr MM, Malhotra V, Briscoe G, Suidan R, Dholakiya P, Santos K, et al. Postoperative pain medication requirements in patients undergoing computer-assisted ("Robotic") and standard laparoscopic procedures for newly diagnosed endometrial cancer. Annals of Surgical Oncology. 2013;**20**(11):3561–3567. DOI: 10.1245/s10434-013-3064-9

[35] Manchana T, Puangsricharoen P, Sirisabya N, Worasethsin P, Vasuratna A, Termrungruanglert W, et al. Comparison of perioperative and oncologic outcomes with laparotomy, and laparoscopic or robotic surgery for women with endometrial cancer. Asian Pacific Journal of Cancer Prevention. 2015;**16**(13):5483–5488. DOI: 10.7314/apjcp.2015.16.13.5483

[36] Mäenpää MM, Nieminen K, Tomás EI, Laurila M, Luukkaala TH, Mäenpää JU. Robotic-assisted vs traditional laparoscopic surgery for endometrial cancer: A randomized controlled trial. American Journal of Obstetrics and Gynecology. 2016;**215**(5):588.e1–.e7. DOI: 10.1016/j.ajog.2016.06.005

[37] Rajadurai VA, Tan J, Salfinger SG, Cohen PA. Outcomes in women undergoing robotic-assisted laparoscopic hysterectomy compared to conventional laparoscopic hysterectomy at a tertiary hospital in Western Australia. Australian & New Zealand Journal of Obstetrics & Gynaecology. 2018;**58**(4):443–448. DOI: 10.1111/ajo.12749

[38] Enes H, Semir I, Sefik H, Husnija M, Goran I. Postoperative pain in open vs. laparoscopic cholecystectomy with and without local application of anaesthetic. Medicinski Glasnik : Official Publication of the Medical Association of Zenica-Doboj Canton, Bosnia and Herzegovina. 2011;**8**(2):243–248

[39] Fu H, Zhang J, Zhao S, He N. Survival outcomes of robotic-assisted laparoscopy versus conventional laparoscopy and laparotomy for endometrial cancer: A systematic review and meta-analysis. Gynecologic Oncology. 2023;**174**:55–67. DOI: 10.1016/j.ygyno.2023.04.026

[40] Eoh KJ, Lee DW, Lee JH, Nam EJ, Kim SW, Kim YT. Comparative survival outcome of robot-assisted staging surgery using three robotic arms versus open surgery for endometrial cancer. Yonsei Medical Journal. 2021;**62**(1):68–74. DOI: 10.3349/ymj.2021.62.1.68

[41] Nicole N, Rachel C, Michael M, Ross B, Sue G, Allison V, et al. Robotic assisted, total laparoscopic, and total abdominal hysterectomy for management of uterine cancer. Journal of Cancer Therapy. 2012;**3**(2):162–166. DOI: 10.4236/jct.2012.32022

[42] Cho SH, Lee JY, Nam EJ, Kim S, Kim YT, Kim SW. Comparison of single-port laparoscopy with other surgical approaches in endometrial cancer surgical staging: Propensity-score-matched analysis. Cancers (Basel). 2023;**15**(22). DOI: 10.3390/cancers15225322

[43] Goel M, Zollinger TW, Moore DH. Surgical staging of endometrial cancer:

Robotic versus open technique outcomes in a contemporary single surgeon series. Journal of Robotic Surgery. 2011;**5**(2):109–114. DOI: 10.1007/s11701-010-0239-2

[44] Bourgin C, Lambaudie E, Houvenaeghel G, Foucher F, Levêque J, Lavoué V. Impact of age on surgical staging and approaches (laparotomy, laparoscopy and robotic surgery) in endometrial cancer management. European Journal of Surgical Oncology (EJSO). 2017;**43**(4):703–709. DOI: 10.1016/j.ejso.2016.10.022

[45] Bell MC, Torgerson J, Seshadri-Kreaden U, Suttle AW, Hunt S. Comparison of outcomes and cost for endometrial cancer staging via traditional laparotomy, standard laparoscopy and robotic techniques. Gynecologic Oncology. 2008;**111** (3):407–411. DOI: 10.1016/j.ygyno.2008.08.022

[46] Silva ESA, de Carvalho JPM, Anton C, Fernandes RP, Baracat EC, Carvalho JP. Introduction of robotic surgery for endometrial cancer into a Brazilian cancer service: A randomized trial evaluating perioperative clinical outcomes and costs. Clinics (Sao Paulo). Clinics. 2018;**73**(suppl 1):e522s. DOI: 10.6061/clinics/2017/e522s

[47] Corrado G, Vizza E, Perrone AM, Mereu L, Cela V, Legge F, et al. Comparison between laparoscopic and robotic surgery in elderly patients with endometrial cancer: A retrospective multicentric study. Frontiers in Oncology. 2021;**11**:724886. DOI: 10.3389/fonc.2021.724886

[48] Perrone E, Capasso I, Pasciuto T, Gioè A, Gueli Alletti S, Restaino S, et al. Laparoscopic vs. robotic-assisted laparoscopy in endometrial cancer staging: Large retrospective single-institution study. Journal of Gynecologic Oncology. 2021;**32**(3):e45. DOI: 10.3802/jgo.2021.32.e45

[49] Jung YW, Lee DW, Kim SW, Nam EJ, Kim JH, Kim JW, et al. Robot-assisted staging using three robotic arms for endometrial cancer: Comparison to laparoscopy and laparotomy at a single institution. Journal of Surgical Oncology. 2010;**101**(2):116–121. DOI: 10.1002/jso.21436

[50] Bogani G, Multinu F, Dowdy SC, Cliby WA, Wilson TO, Gostout BS, et al. Incorporating robotic-assisted surgery for endometrial cancer staging: Analysis of morbidity and costs. Gynecologic Oncology. 2016;**141** (2):218–224. DOI: 10.1016/j.ygyno.2016.02.016

[51] Wright JD, Burke WM, Wilde ET, Lewin SN, Charles AS, Kim JH, et al. Comparative effectiveness of robotic versus laparoscopic hysterectomy for endometrial cancer. Journal of Clinical Oncology. 2012;**30**(8):783–791. DOI: 10.1200/jco.2011.36.7508

[52] Raventós-Tato RM, de la Torre-fernández de Vega J, Sánchez-Iglesias JL, Díaz-Feijoó B, Sabadell J, Pérez-Benavente MA, et al. Surgical approaches in women with endometrial cancer with a body mass index greater than 35 kg/m2. Journal of Obstetrics & Gynaecology Research. 2019;**45**(1):195–202. DOI: 10.1111/jog.13789

[53] Lindfors A, Heshar H, Adok C, Sundfeldt K, Dahm-Kähler P. Long-term survival in obese patients after robotic or open surgery for endometrial cancer. Gynecologic Oncology. 2020;**158**(3):673–680. DOI: 10.1016/j.ygyno.2020.05.684

[54] Mendivil AA, Rettenmaier MA, Abaid LN, Brown 3rd JV, Micha JP, Lopez KL, et al. A comparison of open surgery, robotic-assisted surgery and conventional laparoscopic surgery in the treatment of morbidly obese endometrial cancer patients. Journal of the Society of Laparoendoscopic Surgeons. 2015;**19**(1):e2014.00001. DOI: 10.4293/jsls.2014.00001

[55] Cardenas-Goicoechea J, Soto E, Chuang L, Gretz H, Randall TC. Integration of robotics into two established programs of minimally invasive surgery for endometrial cancer appears to decrease surgical complications. Journal of Gynecologic Oncology. 2013;**24**(1):21–28. DOI: 10.3802/jgo.2013.24.1.21

[56] Boggess JF, Gehrig PA, Cantrell L, Shafer A, Ridgway M, Skinner EN, et al. A comparative study of 3 surgical methods for hysterectomy with staging for endometrial cancer: Robotic assistance, laparoscopy, laparotomy. American Journal of Obstetrics and Gynecology. 2008;**199**(4):360.e1–9. DOI: 10.1016/j.ajog.2008.08.012

[57] Seamon LG, Bryant SA, Rheaume PS, Kimball KJ, Huh WK, Fowler JM, et al. Comprehensive surgical staging for endometrial cancer in obese patients: Comparing robotics and laparotomy. Obstetrics & Gynecology. 2009;**114**(1):16–21. DOI: 10.1097/AOG.0b013e3181aa96c7

[58] Gehrig PA, Cantrell LA, Shafer A, Abaid LN, Mendivil A, Boggess JF. What is the optimal minimally invasive surgical procedure for endometrial cancer staging in the obese and morbidly obese woman? Gynecologic Oncology. 2008;**111**(1):41–45. DOI: 10.1016/j.ygyno.2008.06.030

[59] Beck TL, Schiff MA, Goff BA, Robotic URR. Laparoscopic, or open hysterectomy: Surgical outcomes by approach in endometrial cancer. Journal of Minimally Invasive Gynecology. 2018;**25**(6):986–993. DOI: 10.1016/j.jmig.2018.01.010

[60] ElSahwi KS, Hooper C, De Leon MC, Gallo TN, Ratner E, Silasi DA, et al. Comparison between 155 cases of robotic vs. 150 cases of open surgical staging for endometrial cancer. Gynecologic Oncology. 2012;**124**(2):260–264. DOI: 10.1016/j.ygyno.2011.09.038

[61] Yoshida K, Kondo E, Nimura R, Maki S, Kaneda M, Nii M, et al. Laparoscopic versus robotic hysterectomy in obese patients with early-stage endometrial cancer: A single-centre analysis. Anticancer Research. 2021;**41**(8):4163–4167. DOI: 10.21873/anticanres.15220

[62] Eoh KJ, Kim TJ, Park JY, Kim HS, Paek J, Kim YT. Robot-assisted versus conventional laparoscopic surgery for endometrial cancer: Long-term comparison of outcomes. Frontiers in Oncology. 2023;**13**:1219371. DOI: 10.3389/fonc.2023.1219371

[63] Lundin ES, Wodlin NB, Nilsson L, Kjölhede P. A prospective randomized assessment of quality of life between open and robotic hysterectomy in early endometrial cancer. International Journal of Gynecological Cancer. 2019;**29**:721–727. DOI: 10.1136/ijgc-2019-000285

[64] Park HK, Helenowski IB, Berry E, Lurain JR, Neubauer NL. A comparison of survival and recurrence outcomes in patients with endometrial cancer undergoing robotic versus open surgery.

Journal of Minimally Invasive Gynecology. 2015;**22**(6):961–967. DOI: 10.1016/j.jmig.2015.04.018

[65] Yoon JH, Yun CY, Choi S, Park DC, Kim SI. Is robotic surgery beneficial for the treatment of endometrial cancer? A comparison with conventional laparoscopic surgery. Journal of Cancer. 2024;**15**(2):533–538. DOI: 10.7150/jca.88187

[66] Lim YH, Dagher C, Abu-Rustum NR, Mueller JJ, Sonoda Y, Zivanovic O, et al. Oncologic outcomes of robot-assisted laparoscopy versus conventional laparoscopy for the treatment of apparent early-stage endometrioid adenocarcinoma of the uterus. Gynecologic Oncology. 2023;**179**:152–157

[67] Wright JD, Burke WM, Tergas AI, Hou JY, Huang Y, Hu JC, et al. Comparative Effectiveness of Minimally Invasive Hysterectomy for Endometrial Cancer. Journal of Clinical Oncology. 2016;**34**(10):1087–1096. DOI: 10.1200/jco.2015.65.3212

[68] Estape R, Lambrou N, Estape E, Vega O, Ojea T. Robotic-assisted total laparoscopic hysterectomy and staging for the treatment of endometrial cancer: A comparison with conventional laparoscopy and abdominal approaches. Journal of Robotic Surgery. 2012;**6**(3):199–205. DOI: 10.1007/s11701-011-0290-7

[69] Somashekhar SP, Jaka RC, Zaveri SS. Prospective randomized study comparing robotic-assisted hysterectomy and regional lymphadenectomy with traditional laparotomy for staging of endometrial carcinoma – initial Indian Experience. Indian Journal of Surgical Oncology. 2014;**5**(3):217–223. DOI: 10.1007/s13193-014-0321-8

[70] Cardenas-Goicoechea J, Shepherd A, Momeni M, Mandeli J, Chuang L, Gretz H, et al. Survival analysis of robotic versus traditional laparoscopic surgical staging for endometrial cancer. American Journal of Obstetrics and Gynecology. 2014;**210**(2):160.e1–.e11. DOI: 10.1016/j.ajog.2013.10.871

[71] Agarwal R, Rajanbabu A, Goel G, Unnikrishnan UG. A comparison of the clinical outcomes in uterine cancer surgery after the introduction of robotic-assisted surgery. The Journal of Obstetrics and Gynecology of India. 2019;**69**(3):284–291. DOI: 10.1007/s13224-018-1170-0

[72] Bernardini MQ, Gien LT, Tipping H, Murphy J, Rosen BP. Surgical outcome of robotic surgery in morbidly obese patient with endometrial cancer compared to laparotomy. International Journal of Gynecological Cancer. 2012;**22**(1):76–81. DOI: 10.1097/IGC.0b013e3182353371

[73] Song J, Le T, Hopkins L, Fung-Kee-Fung M, Lupe K, Gaudet M, et al. A comparison of disease recurrence between robotic versus laparotomy approach in patients with intermediate-risk endometrial cancer. International Journal of Gynecological Cancer. 2020;**30**(2):160–166. DOI: 10.1136/ijgc-2019-000838

[74] Bizzarri N, Restaino S, Gueli Alletti S, Monterossi G, Gioè A, La Fera E, et al. Sentinel lymph node detection in endometrial cancer with indocyanine green: Laparoscopic versus robotic approach. Facts, Views and

Vision in ObGyn. 2021;**13**(1):15–25. DOI: 10.52054/fvvo.13.1.002

[75] Renaud MC, Sebastianelli A, Grégoire J, Plante M. Five-year experience in the surgical treatment of endometrial cancer: comparing laparotomy with robotic and minimally invasive hysterectomy. Journal of Obstetrics and Gynaecology Canada. 2022;**44**(1):21–27. DOI: 10.1016/j.jogc.2021.07.021

[76] Chan JK, Gardner AB, Taylor K, Thompson CA, Blansit K, Yu X, et al. Robotic versus laparoscopic versus open surgery in morbidly obese endometrial cancer patients — A comparative analysis of total charges and complication rates. Gynecologic Oncology. 2015;**139**(2):300–305. DOI: 10.1016/j.ygyno.2015.09.006

[77] Corrado G, Cutillo G, Pomati G, Mancini E, Sperduti I, Patrizi L, et al. Surgical and oncological outcome of robotic surgery compared to laparoscopic and abdominal surgery in the management of endometrial cancer. European Journal of Surgical Oncology (EJSO). 2015;**41**(8):1074–1081. DOI: 10.1016/j.ejso.2015.04.020

[78] Magrina JF, Zanagnolo V, Giles D, Noble BN, Kho RM, Magtibay PM. Robotic surgery for endometrial cancer: Comparison of perioperative outcomes and recurrence with laparoscopy, vaginal/laparoscopy and laparotomy. European Journal of Gynaecological Oncology. 2011;**32**(5):476–480

[79] Turunen H, Pakarinen P, Sjöberg J, Loukovaara M. Laparoscopic vs robotic-assisted surgery for endometrial carcinoma in a centre with long laparoscopic experience. Journal of Obstetrics and Gynaecology. 2013;**33**(7):720–724. DOI: 10.3109/01443615.2013.812623

[80] Lim PC, Kang E, Park DH. A comparative detail analysis of the learning curve and surgical outcome for robotic hysterectomy with lymphadenectomy versus laparoscopic hysterectomy with lymphadenectomy in treatment of endometrial cancer: A case-matched controlled study of the first one hundred twenty two patients. Gynecologic Oncology. 2011;**120**(3):413–418. DOI: 10.1016/j.ygyno.2010.11.034

[81] Backes FJ, ElNaggar AC, Farrell MR, Brudie LA, Ahmad S, Salani R, et al. Perioperative outcomes for laparotomy compared to robotic surgical staging of endometrial cancer in the elderly: a retrospective cohort. International Journal of Gynecological Cancer. 2016;**26**(9):1717–1721. DOI: 10.1097/igc.0000000000000822

[82] Johnson L, Bunn WD, Nguyen L, Rice J, Raj M, Cunningham MJ. Clinical comparison of robotic, laparoscopic, and open hysterectomy procedures for endometrial cancer patients. Journal of Robotic Surgery. 2017;**11**(3):291–297. DOI: 10.1007/s11701-016-0651-3

[83] Göçmen A, Sanlıkan F, Uçar MG. Comparison of robotic-assisted surgery outcomes with laparotomy for endometrial cancer staging in Turkey. Archives of Gynecology & Obstetrics. 2010;**282**(5):539–545. DOI: 10.1007/s00404-010-1593-z

[84] Lindfors A, Å Å, Staf C, Sjöli P, Sundfeldt K, Dahm-Kähler P. Robotic vs open surgery for endometrial cancer in elderly patients: Surgical outcome, survival, and cost analysis. International Journal of Gynecological Cancer.

2018;**28**(4):692–699. DOI: 10.1097/igc.0000000000001240

[85] Aiko K, Kanno K, Yanai S, Masuda S, Yasui M, Ichikawa F, et al. Short-term outcomes of robot-assisted versus conventional laparoscopic surgery for early-stage endometrial cancer: A retrospective, single-center study. Journal of Obstetrics & Gynaecology Research. 2020;**46**(7):1157–1164. DOI: 10.1111/jog.14293

[86] Crane EK, Brown J, Lehman A, Tait DL, Naumann RW. Perioperative recovery and narcotic use in laparoscopic versus robotic surgery for endometrial cancer. Journal of Minimally Invasive Gynecology. 2021;**28**(11):1898–1902. DOI: 10.1016/j.jmig.2021.04.022

[87] Hayashi S, Yamanaka Z, Kojima J, Ono M, Sasaki T, Yamamoto A, et al. Retrospective comparative study of robot-assisted surgery, laparoscopic surgery, and laparotomy for endometrial cancer in patients with a low risk of recurrence. Journal of Obstetrics & Gynaecology Research. 2024;**50**(1):103–112. DOI: 10.1111/jog.15816

[88] DeNardis SA, Holloway RW, Bigsby GE, Pikaart DP, Ahmad S, Finkler NJ. Robotically assisted laparoscopic hysterectomy versus total abdominal hysterectomy and lymphadenectomy for endometrial cancer. Gynecologic Oncology. 2008;**111**(3):412–417. DOI: 10.1016/j.ygyno.2008.08.025

[89] Johansson CYM, Chan FKH. Robotic-assisted versus conventional laparoscopic hysterectomy for endometrial cancer. European Journal of Obstetrics & Gynecology and Reproductive Biology: X. 2020;**8**:100116. DOI: 10.1016/j.eurox.2020.100116

[90] Guy MS, Sheeder J, Behbakht K, Wright JD, Guntupalli SR. Comparative outcomes in older and younger women undergoing laparotomy or robotic surgical staging for endometrial cancer. American Journal of Obstetrics and Gynecology. 2016;**214**(3):350.e1–.e10. DOI: 10.1016/j.ajog.2015.09.085

[91] Escobar PF, Frumovitz M, Soliman PT, Frasure HE, Fader AN, Schmeler KM, et al. Comparison of single-port laparoscopy, standard laparoscopy, and robotic surgery in patients with endometrial cancer. Annals of Surgical Oncology. 2012;**19**(5):1583–1588. DOI: 10.1245/s10434-011-2136-y

[92] Lim PC, Kang E, Park DH. Learning curve and surgical outcome for robotic-assisted hysterectomy with lymphadenectomy: Case-matched controlled comparison with laparoscopy and laparotomy for treatment of endometrial cancer. Journal of Minimally Invasive Gynecology. 2010;**17**(6):739–748. DOI: 10.1016/j.jmig.2010.07.008

[93] Cardenas-Goicoechea J, Wang YU, Lee J-H, Shoraka M, Carbajal-Mamani SL, Fishman D, Riner AN, Trevino JG, et al. Survival after minimally invasive surgery in older women with endometrial carcinoma. Anticancer Research. 2022;**42**(1):75–85. DOI: 10.21873/anticanres.15459

[94] Tomov ST, Gorchev GA, Kiprova DK, Lyubenov AD, Hinkova NH, Tomova VD, et al. Peri-operative and survival outcomes analysis of patients with endometrial

cancer managed by three surgical approaches: A long-term Bulgarian experience. Journal of Robotic Surgery. 2022;**16**(6):1367–1382. DOI: 10.1007/s11701-022-01374-0

[95] Seamon LG, Cohn DE, Henretta MS, Kim KH, Carlson MJ, Phillips GS, et al. Minimally invasive comprehensive surgical staging for endometrial cancer: Robotics or laparoscopy? Gynecologic Oncology. 2009;**113**(1):36–41. DOI: 10.1016/j.ygyno.2008.12.005

[96] Doo DW, Guntupalli SR, Corr BR, Sheeder J, Davidson SA, Behbakht K, et al. Comparative surgical outcomes for endometrial cancer patients 65 years old or older staged with robotics or laparotomy. Annals of Surgical Oncology. 2015;**22**(11):3687–3694. DOI: 10.1245/s10434-015-4428-0

[97] Corrado G, Vizza E, Cela V, Mereu L, Bogliolo S, Legge F, et al. Laparoscopic versus robotic hysterectomy in obese and extremely obese patients with endometrial cancer: A multi-institutional analysis. European Journal of Surgical Oncology. 2018;**44**(12):1935–1941. DOI: 10.1016/j.ejso.2018.08.021

[98] Subramaniam A, Kim KH, Bryant SA, Zhang B, Sikes C, Kimball KJ, et al. A cohort study evaluating robotic versus laparotomy surgical outcomes of obese women with endometrial carcinoma. Gynecologic Oncology. 2011;**122**(3):604–607. DOI: 10.1016/j.ygyno.2011.05.024

[99] Eoh KJ, Nam EJ, Kim SW, Shin M, Kim SJ, Kim JA, et al. Nationwide comparison of surgical and oncologic outcomes in endometrial cancer patients undergoing robotic, laparoscopic, and open surgery: a population-based cohort study. Cancer Research and Treatment. 2021;**53**(2):549–557. DOI: 10.4143/crt.2020.802

[100] Chambers LM, Carr C, Freeman L, Jernigan AM, Michener CM. Does surgical platform impact recurrence and survival? A study of utilization of multiport, single-port, and robotic-assisted laparoscopy in endometrial cancer surgery. American Journal of Obstetrics and Gynecology. 2019;**221**(3):243.e1–.e11. DOI: 10.1016/j.ajog.2019.04.038

[101] Hoekstra AV, Jairam-Thodla A, Rademaker A, Singh DK, Buttin BM, Lurain JR, et al. The impact of robotics on practice management of endometrial cancer: Transitioning from traditional surgery. The International Journal of Medical Robotics and Computer Assisted Surgery. 2009;**5**(4):392–397. DOI: 10.1002/rcs.268

[102] El-Achi V, Weishaupt J, Carter J, Saidi S. Robotic versus laparoscopic hysterectomy in morbidly obese women for endometrial cancer. Journal of Robotic Surgery. 2021;**15**(3):483–487. DOI: 10.1007/s11701-020-01133-z

[103] Pant A, Schink J, Lurain J. Robotic surgery compared with laparotomy for high-grade endometrial cancer. Journal of Robotic Surgery. 2014;**8**(2):163–167. DOI: 10.1007/s11701-013-0448-6

[104] Barrie A, Freeman AH, Lyon L, Garcia C, Conell C, Abbott LH, et al. Classification of postoperative complications in robotic-assisted compared with laparoscopic hysterectomy for endometrial cancer. journal of minimally invasive gynecology. 2016;**23**(7):1181–1188. DOI: 10.1016/j.jmig.2016.08.832

[105] Sofer A, Magnezi R, Eitan R, Raban O, Tal O, Smorgic N, et al. Robotic vs. open surgery in obese women with low-grade endometrial cancer: Comparison of costs and quality of life measures. Israel Journal of Health Policy Research. 2020;**9**(1):60. DOI: 10.1186/s13584-020-00412-2

[106] Pakish J, Soliman PT, Frumovitz M, Westin SN, Schmeler KM, Reis RD, et al. A comparison of extraperitoneal versus transperitoneal laparoscopic or robotic para-aortic lymphadenectomy for staging of endometrial carcinoma. Gynecologic Oncology. 2014;**132** (2):366–371. DOI: 10.1016/j.ygyno.2013.12.019

[107] Eklind S, Lindfors A, Sjöli P, Dahm-Kähler P. A prospective, comparative study on roboticversus open-surgery hysterectomy and pelviclymphadenectomy for endometrial carcinoma. International Journal of Gynecological Cancer. 2015;**25**(2):250–256. DOI: 10.1097/igc.0000000000000357

[108] Seror J, Bats AS, Huchon C, Bensaïd C, Douay-Hauser N, Lécuru F. Laparoscopy vs robotics in surgical management of endometrial cancer: Comparison of intraoperative and postoperative complications. Journal of Minimally Invasive Gynecology. 2014;**21**(1):120–125. DOI: 10.1016/j.jmig.2013.07.015

[109] Argenta PA, Mattson J, Rivard CL, Luther E, Schefter A, Vogel RI. Robot-assisted versus laparoscopic minimally invasive surgery for the treatment of stage I endometrial cancer. Gynecologic Oncology. 2022;**165** (2):347–352. DOI: 10.1016/j.ygyno.2022.03.007

[110] Coronado PJ, Herraiz MA, Magrina JF, Fasero M, Vidart JA. Comparison of perioperative outcomes and cost of robotic-assisted laparoscopy, laparoscopy and laparotomy for endometrial cancer. European Journal of Obstetrics & Gynecology and Reproductive Biology. 2012;**165**(2): 289–294. DOI: 10.1016/j.ejogrb.2012.07.006

[111] Safdieh J, Lee YC, Wong A, Lee A, Weiner JP, Schwartz D, et al. A comparison of outcomes between open hysterectomy and robotic-assisted hysterectomy for endometrial cancer using the national cancer database. International Journal of Gynecological Cancer. 2017;**27**(7):1508–1516. DOI: 10.1097/igc.0000000000001034

Section 3

Advances in Thoracic Minimally Invasive Surgery

Chapter 4

Evolution of Minimally Invasive Thoracic Surgery

Ömer Faruk Sağlam

Abstract

Minimally invasive thoracic surgery (MITS) has revolutionized the landscape of thoracic surgical practice, transforming patient care with enhanced precision and reduced invasiveness. This chapter chronicles the evolutionary journey of MITS, from its nascent stages with early thoracoscopic techniques to the widespread adoption of advanced video-assisted thoracoscopic surgery (VATS) and robotic-assisted thoracic surgery (RATS). We delve into pivotal technological advancements, including high-definition imaging, sophisticated endoscopic instrumentation, and cutting-edge robotic platforms, which have been instrumental in redefining surgical paradigms and improving patient outcomes. Furthermore, the chapter explores current global trends, the complexities of training and adoption, and offers a forward-looking perspective on emerging technologies, including artificial intelligence, augmented reality, and soft robotics. This comprehensive overview aims to provide surgeons, trainees, and innovators with a profound understanding of the trajectory and immense potential of minimally invasive approaches to thoracic surgery.

Keywords: video-assisted thoracic surgery, robotic-assisted thoracic surgery, minimally invasive thoracic surgery, surgical innovation, minimally invasive techniques

1. Introduction

Minimally invasive thoracic surgery (MITS) represents a paradigm shift in the surgical management of thoracic diseases, moving away from traditional open procedures that necessitated large incisions and significant disruption of the chest wall. This evolution has been driven by a relentless pursuit of improved patient outcomes, characterized by reduced post-operative pain, shorter hospital stays, faster recovery times, and enhanced cosmetic results. The advent of MITS has not only transformed the technical aspects of thoracic operations but has also profoundly influenced clinical decision-making, patient selection, and the overall trajectory of care for a wide spectrum of conditions affecting the lungs, mediastinum, esophagus, and chest wall.

Historically, thoracic surgery was synonymous with extensive open thoracotomies procedures that, while effective, were associated with considerable morbidity, including severe pain, prolonged recovery, and potential complications such as chronic post-thoracotomy pain syndrome. The inherent invasiveness of these traditional approaches often limited their applicability, particularly in frail or elderly patients, and imposed a significant burden on healthcare resources due to extended hospitalization and rehabilitation needs. The imperative to mitigate these drawbacks has spurred innovation, leading to the gradual development and refinement of less invasive techniques.

This chapter aims to provide a comprehensive exploration of the evolution of MITS, tracing its origins from rudimentary endoscopic observations to sophisticated robotic platforms available today. We delineate the key milestones that have shaped this transformative journey, highlighting the technological breakthroughs that have enabled surgeons to perform complex procedures through small incisions with unprecedented precision. A significant portion of this discussion will be dedicated to understanding the impact of video-assisted thoracoscopic surgery (VATS) and robotic-assisted thoracic surgery (RATS), two cornerstones of modern MITS, on surgical practice and patient care. Furthermore, we will examine the current global landscape of MITS adoption, the challenges associated with training and implementation, and offer an insightful outlook on the future directions of this dynamic field, including the integration of artificial intelligence (AI), augmented reality (AR), and soft robotics. By chronicling this evolution, we seek to provide valuable resources for surgeons, trainees, and innovators who are committed to advancing the frontiers of thoracic surgical care.

2. Historical development of minimally invasive thoracic surgery

2.1. Early thoracoscopy and its pioneers

The concept of visualizing internal body cavities without large incisions dates back to the early twentieth century, laying the groundwork for what would eventually become minimally invasive surgery. While the widespread adoption of thoracoscopy in thoracic surgery is a relatively recent phenomenon, its origins are traditionally attributed to Hans Christian Jacobaeus, who, in 1910, utilized a rigid cystoscope to perform diagnostic and therapeutic thoracoscopy in patients with tuberculous pleuritis, thereby establishing the foundation for modern thoracoscopic surgery [1]. However, a historical reassessment presented by Gordon and later discussed by Migliore suggests that the first documented thoracoscopic procedure may, in fact, predate Jacobaeus. In 1866, Sir Francis Richard Cruise of Dublin performed pleural endoscopy on a young female patient with hydrothorax. Using a modified version of a Desormeaux endoscope, Cruise inserted the instrument into the pleural cavity through a trocar to visualize the internal pathology. His intervention, although not formally recognized in surgical literature for decades, was documented in hospital records and later analyzed by Gordon [2]. In light of this historical evidence and in the absence of any prior published cases, it is justifiable to credit Sir Francis Richard Cruise as the first physician to have conducted documented thoracoscopy. Nevertheless, Jacobaeus systematically described the procedure and catalyzed its integration into clinical practice, securing his place as the pivotal figure in the emergence of thoracoscopy in the twentieth century.

Early thoracoscopy was primarily employed in the context of tuberculosis treatment, specifically for pneumothorax induction and adhesiolysis to facilitate lung collapse. The instruments available were primitive by today's standards, consisting of rigid endoscopes with limited illumination and no video capabilities. Surgeons had to peer directly through the scope, often in dimly lit operating rooms, making the procedures technically challenging and restricting their scope to relatively simple interventions. The lack of adequate visualization and instrumentation meant that complex resections or intricate dissections were beyond the realm of possibility. Furthermore, the absence of effective hemostatic tools posed significant risks, limiting the procedures to those with minimal bleeding potential.

Despite these limitations, other early pioneers, such as Janos Hellinger and Richard W. Light, established the foundational principles of thoracoscopy. They demonstrated the feasibility of accessing the pleural space and performing certain procedures with less invasiveness than traditional open surgery. However, the inherent challenges of direct-view endoscopy, including a restricted field of vision, poor illumination, and the inability to share the surgical view with assistants, have prevented thoracoscopy from gaining widespread acceptance as a primary surgical approach. For decades, it has remained a niche procedure, largely confined to specialized centers and primarily used for diagnostic purposes or minor therapeutic interventions in select cases of pleural disease.

The technological constraints of this era were significant impediments to the broader application of thoracoscopy. The rigid endoscopes offered a narrow, two-dimensional view, and the illumination provided by small incandescent bulbs or external light sources was often insufficient for clear visualization of the thoracic cavity. The instruments used for manipulation and dissection were cumbersome and lacked the precision and articulation required for complex surgical tasks. Moreover, the absence of video technology meant that the surgeon was the sole observer, making teaching and collaborative surgery difficult. These factors collectively contributed to the slow evolution of thoracoscopy and its limited role in mainstream thoracic surgery for much of the twentieth century. The stage was set for a technological revolution that would fundamentally alter the landscape of thoracic surgical practice. However, for the next several decades, thoracoscopy remained limited in scope. It was largely relegated to diagnostic inspection of the pleural space and simple interventions such as pleural biopsy or adhesiolysis in benign conditions, while major intrathoracic operations still required open thoracotomy. Technical constraints of the era – dim lighting, primitive optics, and lack of instruments to securely address sizable intrathoracic structures – confined thoracoscopy to a supportive role.

2.2. The advent of video-assisted thoracoscopic surgery (VATS)

The true revolution in MITS began with the advent of VATS in the early 1990s. This transformative shift was primarily driven by significant advancements in video technology, particularly the development of small, high-resolution cameras coupled with fiber-optic light sources. These innovations have allowed for a magnified, illuminated, and, most importantly, projected view of the surgical field onto a monitor, fundamentally changing the dynamics of thoracic surgery [3]. The ability to visualize the internal anatomy on a screen not only improved clarity and detail but also enabled the entire surgical team to observe the procedure simultaneously, facilitating collaboration and enhancing the learning process for trainees.

The first successful VATS lobectomy was performed by Giancarlo Roviaro in Milan, Italy, in 1991 [4]. This landmark event marked a pivotal moment, demonstrating the feasibility and safety of performing major thoracic resections through small incisions without the need for a large thoracotomy. Following this pioneering work, VATS rapidly gained traction, with numerous centers worldwide adopting and refining the technique for a wide array of thoracic pathologies, including lung cancer, mediastinal tumors, and pleural diseases.

Initially, VATS procedures were typically performed using multiple small incisions (ports), ranging from two to four, to introduce the camera and various surgical instruments. This multi-port approach allowed for triangulation of instruments, providing surgeons with a familiar operative setup akin to open surgery, albeit through smaller access points. Over time, as surgical expertise grew and instrumentation became more sophisticated, there was a gradual evolution toward fewer ports. This culminated in the development and increasing adoption of uniportal VATS (UVATS), where all instruments and the camera are introduced through a single small incision, typically in the range of 3–5 cm [5]. UVATS further minimizes surgical trauma, potentially leading to even less post-operative pain and faster recovery, although it presents a steeper learning curve for surgeons due to the lack of triangulation [6–8].

The advantages of VATS over traditional open thoracotomy quickly became evident and were substantiated by a growing body of clinical evidence. Patients undergoing VATS experienced significantly reduced post-operative pain, largely due to the avoidance of rib spreading and muscle division inherent in open procedures. This reduction in pain translated to a decreased need for opioid analgesics and facilitated earlier mobilization. Furthermore, VATS was associated with shorter hospital stays, faster recovery times, and a quicker return to normal activities [9–11]. The smaller incisions also resulted in improved cosmetic outcomes, which, while not directly impacting clinical recovery, contributed to patient satisfaction [12]. From an oncological perspective, studies demonstrated that VATS for early-stage lung cancer achieved comparable, if not superior, oncological outcomes to open surgery, including similar rates of complete resection and long-term survival [13]. These compelling benefits solidified VATS's position as the preferred approach for many thoracic surgical procedures, marking a significant leap forward in the evolution of minimally invasive techniques.

2.3. The rise of robotic-assisted thoracic surgery (RATS)

Building upon the foundations laid by VATS, the next significant leap in MITS came with the introduction and widespread adoption of RATS. The development of robotic surgical systems, most notably the da Vinci Surgical System, marked a new era of precision and control in the operating room. While the initial applications of robotic surgery were predominantly in urology and gynecology, its benefits soon became apparent for complex thoracic procedures, leading to its gradual integration into the thoracic surgeon's armamentarium [14].

The da Vinci system, first cleared by the FDA in 2000, offered several distinct advantages over conventional VATS. Key among these was the enhanced three-dimensional (3D) high-definition (HD) visualization, which provided surgeons with an immersive and magnified view of the surgical field, far superior to the 2D monitors used in traditional VATS. This improved depth perception and clarity were crucial for intricate dissections and precise tissue manipulation in the confined space of the thoracic cavity. Furthermore, the robotic instruments, known as EndoWrist instruments, mimicked the dexterity and range of motion of the human wrist, but with a greater degree of articulation (seven degrees of freedom) and tremor filtration. This allowed surgeons to perform delicate maneuvers with unparalleled precision, even in deep and difficult-to-reach anatomical areas [15].

Another significant benefit of RATS is the ergonomic advantage it offers to surgeons. Unlike VATS, in which surgeons often operate in awkward positions, RATS allows the surgeon to sit comfortably at a console, controlling the robotic arms with intuitive hand movements. This reduces physical fatigue during long procedures and can potentially extend the surgeon's career. The system also provides a stable platform, eliminating physiological tremors, which is particularly advantageous for microdissections and suturing in challenging anatomical locations.

Early applications of RATS in thoracic surgery primarily focused on thymectomies, mediastinal tumor resections, and non-anatomic lung resections, where enhanced dexterity and visualization proved particularly beneficial [16]. As surgeons gained experience and confidence, the indications for RATS expanded to include more complex pulmonary resections, such as lobectomies and segmentectomies for lung cancer. Studies have demonstrated that RATS for lung cancer is oncologically sound, with comparable or even superior outcomes to VATS and open surgery in terms of lymph node dissection, margin status, and long-term survival [17].

Despite its numerous advantages, the adoption of RATS has faced certain challenges, primarily related to its high initial cost, the need for specialized training, and a steep learning curve. The capital investment for a robotic system is substantial, and the ongoing costs are associated with maintenance and disposable instruments. However, as the technology continues to evolve and become more accessible, and as the long-term benefits in terms of patient outcomes and reduced complications become more widely recognized, RATS is increasingly becoming a standard of care in many advanced thoracic surgical centers worldwide. This increase signifies a crucial step in the ongoing evolution of MITS, pushing the boundaries of what is surgically possible with minimal patient impact.

Table 1 summarizes a chronological overview of key milestones.

3. Technological advancements and shifting clinical paradigms

The evolution of MITS has been inextricably linked to, and propelled by, a continuous stream of technological advancements. These innovations have not only refined existing techniques but have also fundamentally shifted clinical paradigms, expanding the indications for MITS and improving patient outcomes. From enhanced visualization to sophisticated instrumentation and advanced robotic platforms, technological leaps have contributed to making complex thoracic procedures safer, more precise, and less invasive.

Year	Milestone/innovation
1865	Sir Francis Richard Cruise performed the first thoracoscopy in humans in 1865, overlooking the pleural cavity of a patient with a pleuro-cutaneous fistula.
1910	Jacobaeus performs the first thoracoscopic procedure using a cystoscope in pleural TB.
1920s–1950s	Thoracoscopy is used in Europe for TB and pleural diseases.
1970s	Rigid thoracoscopy explored. Fiberoptic scopes and staplers spur renewed thoracoscopy use, especially in pleural biopsies and talc pleurodesis.
1980s	Video technology enables monitor-based surgery. Early thoracoscopic lung resections were attempted. Gordon and Cruise's thoracoscopic attempts were retrospectively noted.
1991	Roviaro performs first VATS lobectomy in Milan; proves feasibility of thoracoscopic major lung resections.
Mid-1990s	Multi-port VATS techniques develop. VATS is adopted for wedge resections, pleurodesis, and biopsies. Retrospective studies show less pain and faster recovery compared to open surgery.
2000	da Vinci System FDA-approved for surgery; robotic 3D view and wristed instruments raise interest in thoracic use.
2001–2002	Melfi et al. and others published early robotic lung resections, proving RATS feasibility. Early RATS thymectomy and mediastinal mass resections were performed.
2003	Robotic lobectomy introduced
2006–2010	VATS lobectomy is gaining evidence and acceptance. MITS is recommended for early-stage lung cancer.
2010	González-Rivas pioneers uniportal VATS; a single small incision further reduces trauma.
Early 2010s	RATS adopted more widely. RATS ~10–15% of MITS cases. Meta-analyses show comparable or better outcomes than VATS.
2014	ICG fluorescence imaging was adopted for segmentectomy and lymph node mapping.
2016	Robotic sleeve resections demonstrate the applicability of RATS to complex oncological cases. Widespread adoption of robotic platforms is evident in high-volume centers.
2017	Trials begin comparing RATS vs. VATS with high-level evidence. Use of robotic staplers and integrated consoles expands.
2018	Medtronic Hugo and CMR Versius robots launched; they aim to improve access and lower costs.
2019	First 5G-telementored robotic lung surgeries performed across long distances.
2020s	AI, 3D reconstruction, AR, and fluorescence enhance guidance and precision in MITS. Global expansion of RATS; training curricula formalized. Uniportal RATS.
2023–2025	Haptic feedback introduced (e.g., Riverfield Saroa, da Vinci 5 with force-feedback; integration with AR/AI and telesurgery). Single-port and flexible robots developed.

Table 1.
Timeline of MITS milestones [1, 2, 4, 18–32].

3.1. Imaging technologies

Central to the success of MITS is its ability to visualize the surgical field with clarity and detail. Early thoracoscopy was hampered by poor illumination and limited resolution, but modern imaging technologies have overcome these limitations, providing surgeons with an unprecedented view of thoracic anatomy. The transition from standard definition to HD and 3D imaging is a significant milestone. HD cameras offer superior resolution, allowing for the precise identification of anatomical structures and subtle pathological changes. 3D imaging, by providing depth perception, greatly enhances a surgeon's spatial orientation and hand-eye coordination, particularly during complex dissections and suturing, thereby reducing the learning curve for MITS procedures [33].

Advancements in imaging have introduced real-time functional techniques into thoracic surgery, with indocyanine green (ICG) fluorescence emerging as a widely adopted tool. Intravenous ICG highlights vascular and lymphatic structures, aiding in segmental plane identification, anastomotic integrity assessment, and detection of metastatic nodes [5, 34–36]. Beyond pulmonary resections, it has proven useful in evaluating gastric conduit perfusion and thoracic duct ligation [37]. ICG also enhances sentinel lymph node mapping, improving staging accuracy, particularly where nodal involvement is unclear [38], and has been effective in detecting small pulmonary nodules and mesotheliomas [39]. While generally safe, ICG use requires caution in patients with hepatic or renal dysfunction, and its efficacy may be limited in poorly perfused tumors [40, 41]. Fluorescence imaging has also reduced chyle leak rates by improving thoracic duct visualization, though precision is essential to avoid inadvertent injury [42]. Successful integration depends on adequate training and familiarity with fluorescence systems, as emphasized by [43]. ICG fluorescence imaging supports safer, more accurate thoracic surgery, particularly in the context of minimally invasive and anatomically tailored approaches [36].

Furthermore, the integration of navigation systems into MITS is revolutionizing surgical planning and execution. These systems, often based on pre-operative CT scans, create a virtual map of the patient's anatomy. During surgery, instruments can be tracked in real time on this virtual map, guiding the surgeon to target lesions with greater accuracy, especially for small or deeply located nodules that may be difficult to palpate or visualize directly [44]. This fusion of pre-operative imaging with intraoperative navigation enhances precision, particularly in procedures such as segmentectomy, where precise identification of segmental boundaries is crucial.

3.2. Advanced endoscopic instrumentation

The efficacy and safety of MITS rely heavily on the sophistication of the instruments used within the confined thoracic cavity. Over the years, there has been a remarkable evolution in endoscopic instrumentation, transforming from basic grasping and cutting tools to highly specialized devices that mimic the functionality of traditional open surgical instruments, but with the added advantage of being able to operate through small ports. This continuous refinement has been crucial in enabling surgeons to perform increasingly complex procedures with greater precision and control.

One of the most significant advancements in MITS has been the development of advanced energy devices. Instruments such as the Harmonic Scalpel (Ethicon) and LigaSure (Medtronic) enable simultaneous cutting and coagulation through ultrasonic and bipolar energy modalities, respectively, significantly reducing blood loss and operative time. The Harmonic Scalpel operates via high-frequency mechanical vibration and is particularly effective in soft tissue dissection with minimal thermal spread [45], while LigaSure provides reliable vessel sealing for vessels up to 7 mm with integrated feedback control [46]. These technologies have proven especially beneficial in lobectomies and segmentectomies, where precise hemostasis is critical. The THUNDERBEAT system (Olympus), which combines ultrasonic and advanced bipolar energy in a single instrument, has further improved intraoperative efficiency by enabling multi-functionality and reducing instrument exchange [47]. The continuous evolution of these devices has focused on improving safety profiles, minimizing lateral thermal injury, and enhancing ergonomic control to support surgeon precision during thoracic procedures [48].

Modern endoscopic staplers have become essential in MITS, offering enhanced articulation, powered firing, and feedback systems. Devices like Echelon Flex™, Tri-Staple™, and Signia™ improve precision and safety in complex resections. Echelon Flex™ enables better access with 45° articulation and real-time compression feedback, resulting in high surgeon satisfaction and reduced complications [49]. Tri-Staple™ adapts to tissue thickness via graduated staple heights, enhancing hemostasis and reducing bleeding [50]. Signia™ adjusts firing based on tissue resistance, minimizing misfires and improving staple consistency. Clinical studies associate powered staplers with fewer complications, shorter hospital stays, and greater cost-efficiency [51, 52]. These advances mark a shift toward greater precision and reliability in thoracic surgical stapling. Such innovations ensure reliable closure of bronchi and pulmonary vessels, reduce air leaks, and contribute to safer resections in VATS and RATS procedures [5].

The development of specialized tools for specific MITS procedures has also been a key area of innovation. This includes instruments designed for tissue retraction, knot tying, and needle handling, all adapted for endoscopic use. For example, specialized retractors that can be deployed through small ports provide adequate exposure without the need for large incisions. Similarly, advanced needle drivers and knot pushers have made intracorporeal suturing and knot tying more feasible and efficient, thereby reducing reliance on extracorporeal knot tying, which can be less precise.

The trend toward single-port instruments represents another significant leap. While multi-port VATS remains common, the increasing adoption of UVATS has driven the demand for instruments that can be manipulated effectively through a single small incision. This has led to the development of curved instruments, articulating instruments, and instruments with flexible shafts that allow for a wider range of motion and better triangulation within the single port. These innovations aim to further reduce surgical trauma and improve cosmetic outcomes, pushing the boundaries of minimally invasive approaches even further [33]. The continuous innovation in endoscopic instrumentation underscores the commitment to making MITS procedures safer, more efficient, and accessible to a wider range of patients.

3.3. Robotic platforms and their evolution

The evolution of robotic platforms has been a transformative force in MITS, building upon the advantages of VATS and addressing some of its inherent limitations. The da Vinci surgical system, initially developed for military applications, has become the dominant robotic platform in surgery, and its successive generations have significantly refined the capabilities of RATS [15].

The first generation of robotic systems, while revolutionary, had certain limitations, including a lack of haptic feedback (the sensation of touch or force), which meant that surgeons relied solely on visual cues. However, even these early systems offered superior 3D visualization and enhanced dexterity compared to conventional VATS, making complex procedures more manageable. The fixed fulcrum effect of the robotic arms, where the instrument pivots at the port site, also provided a stable platform for precise movements.

Subsequent generations of robotic systems have introduced significant improvements. The da Vinci Si and Xi systems, for instance, brought enhanced ergonomics, improved instrument articulation, and greater flexibility in port placement. The Xi system, with its overhead instrument arm architecture, allows for multi-quadrant access without redocking, making it particularly versatile for complex thoracic procedures that may span different areas of the chest. These advancements have made robotic surgery more efficient and adaptable to a wider range of surgical scenarios [17].

One of the most anticipated advancements in robotic surgery is the integration of haptic feedback technology, which aims to restore tactile sensation by enabling surgeons to perceive tissue resistance and tension during procedures. Although not yet standard across all commercial systems, this capability is now being realized in the da Vinci 5, FDA-approved in 2024 and expected to see widespread adoption by 2026 [24, 29]. Previous robotic platforms lacked tactile feedback, forcing reliance on visual cues, which could limit precision in complex dissections [53, 54]. The incorporation of force-feedback has been shown to improve surgical performance by reducing tissue trauma and enhancing instrument control [28, 55, 56]. In training settings, haptics may also shorten learning curves by simulating realistic tissue interactions [57, 58]. Complementing this, tremor filtration, an intrinsic feature of robotic systems, eliminates involuntary hand movements, enabling ultraprecise tasks such as microdissections and vascular anastomoses. Together, these innovations promise to elevate both the safety and intuitiveness of RATS, marking a significant leap forward in surgical fidelity and ergonomics.

Beyond the da Vinci platform, several next-generation robotic systems have emerged, each offering unique features and clinical advantages. These include platforms with single-port access, advanced imaging integration, and compatibility with AI and AR, all designed to improve precision and decision-making in minimally invasive procedures. Among these, the CMR Versius® system presents a modular and portable alternative, featuring independent bedside units and an open console that facilitate flexibility in operating room setup [59, 60]. Clinical studies have shown Versius achieves comparable outcomes, particularly in colorectal surgery, with reduced conversion rates and a shorter learning curve [61, 62]. In contrast, the da Vinci Xi and SP systems remain benchmarks in robotic surgery, offering HD 3D imaging, tremor filtration, and wristed instruments that enhance dexterity in confined spaces [63–65]. Benefits of the da Vinci system include shorter hospital stays and fewer post-operative complications, though operative times may be longer than conventional methods [66]. While da Vinci emphasizes structured training and comprehensive visual feedback, Versius focuses on ergonomic ease and operational simplicity, promoting quicker adaptation by surgical teams [59, 67]. As robotic platforms continue to evolve toward smaller, smarter, and more versatile designs, they are expected to further transform MITS by making complex procedures achievable through minimal incisions with enhanced precision and control.

3.4. Impact on patient outcomes and surgical practice

The cumulative effect of advancements in imaging technologies, endoscopic instrumentation, and robotic platforms has profoundly impacted both patient outcomes and the fundamental practice of thoracic surgery. The shift from open thoracotomy to minimally invasive approaches, particularly VATS and RATS, has ushered in an era of enhanced patient recovery, reduced morbidity, and expanded surgical capabilities.

One of the most significant and consistently reported benefits of MITS is its reduced invasiveness, which directly translates to less post-operative pain. By avoiding large incisions, rib spreading, and extensive muscle dissection, MITS significantly mitigates the tissue trauma associated with open surgery. This reduction in pain leads to decreased reliance on opioid analgesics, fewer pain-related complications, and a more comfortable recovery experience for patients. Consequently, patients undergoing MITS typically experience shorter hospital stays and are often discharged earlier than those undergoing open procedures. This not only improves patient satisfaction but also contributes to significant cost savings for healthcare systems [44].

Furthermore, reduced surgical trauma associated with MITS facilitates faster recovery and an earlier return to normal activities, including work and daily routines [68]. In a randomized trial, Bendixen et al. demonstrated that VATS lobectomy significantly accelerated functional recovery compared to open thoracotomy, with lower rates of moderate-to-severe pain at 24 hours (38% vs. 63%; $p = 0.0012$), shorter duration of epidural analgesia (median 2 vs. 3 days; $p = 0.022$), and improved quality of life scores during the first year (EQ5D; $p = 0.014$) [69]. These short-term benefits were also reflected in a reduced median hospital stay (4 vs. 5 days; $p = 0.027$). Importantly, long-term outcomes similarly favored VATS; Oda et al. reported significantly higher 5-year overall survival (100% vs. 87%; $p = 0.01$) and disease-free survival (100% vs. 86%; $p = 0.03$) in patients with stage IA NSCLC, along with decreased post-operative inflammation (peak CRP 5.6 vs. 7.9 mg/dL; $p = 0.01$) and shorter chest tube duration (3 vs. 4 days; $p = 0.01$) [70]. Collectively, these findings support the conclusion that minimized access trauma through MITS promotes both rapid convalescence and durable functional outcomes. This is particularly advantageous for patients with comorbidities or those requiring timely adjuvant therapies, as it allows for earlier initiation of post-operative treatments [68, 70]. Additionally, the smaller incisions inherent to MITS offer improved cosmetic results, which, while not directly impacting oncological outcomes, may significantly enhance psychological well-being and body image in the post-operative period [69].

Beyond these immediate benefits, MITS has demonstrated enhanced precision and safety. Magnified, HD visualization provided by video and robotic systems allows surgeons to identify anatomical structures with greater clarity and perform dissections with meticulous accuracy. The articulated instruments of robotic systems, coupled with tremor filtration, enable fine movements and precise suturing in confined spaces, potentially reducing the risk of complications such as bleeding or nerve injury. This heightened precision is particularly crucial in oncological resections, where clear surgical margins and thorough lymph node dissection are paramount for optimal long-term outcomes [17].

The success and safety of MITS have also led to a significant expansion of the indications for minimally invasive approaches. Procedures once considered exclusively within the domain of open surgery, such as complex lung resections (e.g., segmentectomies), mediastinal tumor excisions, and even some esophageal procedures, are now routinely performed using VATS or RATS. This expansion means that more patients, including those who might have been deemed too frail for traditional open surgery, can now benefit from surgical intervention with a lower-risk profile. The ability to offer less invasive options has broadened the patient population eligible for curative or palliative surgical treatment, thereby improving access to care and overall public health outcomes.

In summary, the continuous technological advancements in MITS have not merely refined surgical techniques; they have fundamentally reshaped the landscape of thoracic surgery, prioritizing patient well-being through reduced invasiveness, accelerated recovery, and enhanced surgical precision. This ongoing evolution continues to redefine the standards of care, making thoracic surgery safer, more effective, and more patient-centric.

Comparative domains are outlined in **Table 2**.

Aspect	VATS	RATS
Visualization	2D/HD view, limited depth	3D magnified view
Dexterity	Rigid instruments, limited freedom	Wristed instruments, full range
Tremor handling	No tremor filtering	Tremor eliminated
Haptic feedback	Yes (limited tactile)	Yes
Surgeon ergonomics	Bedside standing, awkward posture, higher fatigue risk	Console-seated; ergonomic setup reduces fatigue
Operative time	Generally shorter with experience	Slightly longer early on; similar after the learning curve
Blood loss	Moderate; depends on the case and technique	Often reduced due to stable control and precision
Conversion to open	5–15% depends on pathology and experience	Lower (~3–5%) with better visualization and control
Complication rate	Comparable to open surgery; reduced in experienced hands.	Equal or lower than VATS in some studies
Length of stay (LOS)	4–6 days on average	3–5 days; potentially shorter with ERAS protocols
Oncological lymph node dissection	Adequate; may vary by surgeon or approach	Higher mediastinal node yield in some series
30-day mortality	1–2%, varies with comorbidities	Comparable or slightly lower in high-volume centers
Pain and recovery	Reduced vs. open; may still have intercostal pain	Lower post-operative pain; less trauma
Cost	Lower per-case and maintenance costs	Higher cost, but long-term cost-effectiveness debated
Learning curve	30–50 cases to proficiency	20–30 cases; dual-console aids training
Technical limitations	Limited flexibility and reach in deep spaces	Larger setup; docking time; assistant dependence

Table 2.
Comparative summary of VATS versus RATS [19, 23, 24, 26, 29, 56, 71–76].

4. Current global trends, training, and barriers to adoption

The widespread adoption of MITS has not been uniform across the world. While the clinical benefits of VATS and RATS are well-established, their integration into routine surgical practice is influenced by a complex interplay of economic, cultural, educational, and infrastructural factors. Understanding these trends, nuances of training, and persistent barriers to adoption is crucial for fostering equitable access to advanced thoracic surgical care worldwide.

4.1. Global adoption rates and regional variations

The prevalence of VATS and RATS varies significantly across regions and countries. Developed nations, particularly in North America, Western Europe, and parts of Asia (e.g., Japan and South Korea), have seen rapid and extensive adoption of MITS, with VATS becoming the standard of care for many lung resections and RATS gaining increasing traction. In these regions, the availability of advanced surgical equipment, robust healthcare infrastructure, and established training programs has facilitated this transition [33]. For instance, in the United States, the proportion of minimally invasive lobectomies has steadily increased, often exceeding 50% in high-volume centers. Moreover, in stage II non-small cell lung cancer (NSCLC), minimally invasive lobectomy can be successfully completed without conversion in approximately 80% of cases, reflecting increased surgical confidence and technical feasibility in managing more advanced disease stages [77].

Despite the global rise of MITS, its adoption remains uneven due to a complex interplay of economic, infrastructural, and cultural factors. Adoption rates in many developing countries remain lower [22]. This disparity can be attributed to several factors. By the mid-2010s, VATS lobectomy had become the standard of care for early-stage lung cancer in many high-income nations; however, utilization rates varied widely – approximately 30–40% in the United States, 30% across most of Europe, with notable outliers such as Denmark (~65%) and Italy (~50%), while countries like the UK reported less than 30% [78]. These discrepancies reflect differences in surgeon training, national policies, and institutional referral patterns. In lower-resource settings, adoption is further constrained by the high upfront investment in equipment (e.g., video towers, specialized or robotic systems), recurring costs for disposables, and limited operating room infrastructure and staffing. Cultural resistance to shifting away from traditional open techniques also plays a role. Nevertheless, multiple studies have demonstrated that after the initial learning curve, RATS achieves comparable operative times and costs to VATS, while preserving its added benefits in dexterity and visualization. These findings, observed across diverse healthcare systems, reinforce that robotic platforms – despite initial barriers – are a sustainable and forward-looking choice for long-term integration in thoracic surgical practice [26, 75, 79].

A regional breakdown of MITS usage is presented in **Table 3**.

Cultural factors and established surgical traditions can also influence the pace of adoption, with some regions being more resistant to rapid changes in surgical practices. Healthcare infrastructure limitations, such as inadequate operating room facilities, insufficient support staff, and unreliable supply chains for specialized equipment, further impede the widespread implementation of MITS [5].

Region	MITS adoption rate (approx.)	Observations and trends
North America	~50% lobectomies via MITS (VATS/RATS)	U.S. saw VATS at ~35% in the 2010s; RATS rose to ~15% by 2015. Some centers exceed 60% MITS. Smaller/rural centers still prefer thoracotomy.
Europe	~30–40% average (Western Europe higher)	Western/Nordic Europe: 40–60% MITS in top centers. Poland: VATS ~35–40% by 2017. RATS growing slowly. ETS efforts ongoing.
Asia-Pacific	~40–60% (high variation by country)	China ~48% (14–75% by region); Japan/Korea have high VATS, with rising RATS after 2018 coverage. Southeast Asia is growing, though there are some limits in access.
Latin America	~20–30% overall (higher in select centers)	Brazil (selected centers): MITS up to 89% by 2020. Public sector use remains low. RATS are rare, mostly in Brazil and Colombia.
Africa and Middle East	<10% overall	Africa: very limited MITS; mainly thoracotomy. Middle East: gradual growth in Turkey, UAE, Israel, and Saudi Arabia. RATS is rare, limited to high-end centers.

Table 3.
Global adoption of MITS by region [20, 22, 33, 77, 78].

Despite these challenges, there is a growing global trend toward increasing MITS adoption, driven by rising awareness of its patient benefits and efforts by international surgical societies to promote training and knowledge transfer. Collaborative initiatives, proctoring programs, and the development of more affordable technologies are gradually bridging the gap between high- and low-income countries, albeit at a slower pace.

4.2. Training and education in MITS

The successful integration of MITS into surgical practice hinges critically on effective training and education. Both VATS and RATS require a distinct skill set that differs significantly from that of traditional open surgery, necessitating specialized training programs to ensure surgeon proficiency and patient safety. The learning curve for these techniques can be steep, particularly for complex procedures, making structured educational pathways essential.

Simulation-based training has emerged as a cornerstone of MITS education. High-fidelity simulators, both virtual reality (VR) and physical models, allow trainees to practice fundamental skills and entire procedures in a risk-free environment. These simulators provide immediate feedback on performance, helping surgeons develop hand-eye coordination, depth perception, and instrument manipulation skills specific to endoscopic and robotic platforms. Simulation training can significantly shorten the initial learning curve and improve confidence before operating on live patients [33].

Beyond simulations, fellowship programs and structured curricula are vital for comprehensive MITS training. These programs typically involve a combination of didactic lectures, hands-on cadaveric or animal lab experience, observation by experienced surgeons, and supervised operative experience. Mentorship from seasoned MITS surgeons is invaluable, as it provides guidance on patient selection, surgical planning, troubleshooting intraoperative challenges, and managing post-operative complications. Structured training initiatives, such as the joint European Society of Thoracic Surgeons–European Respiratory Society curriculum for MITS and the Society of Thoracic Surgeons expert consensus statement on a standardized national robotic curriculum, represent critical steps toward harmonizing skills acquisition and facilitating broader, evidence-based adoption of minimally invasive approaches in thoracic surgery [80, 81].

The learning curves for VATS and RATS are well-documented and represent a significant consideration in training. For VATS lobectomy, studies suggest that a surgeon may need to perform 30–50 cases to achieve proficiency and consistent outcomes comparable to open surgery [44]. The learning curve for RATS is often considered steeper due to the complexity of the robotic platform and the need to master console navigation, multi-joint instrument articulation, and immersive 3D visualization. Proficiency in RATS is estimated to require 20–80 cases, depending on the procedure's complexity and the surgeon's prior MITS experience [17]. However, robotic surgery training offers unique pedagogical advantages not present in VATS, such as dual-console systems, which allow real-time hands-on mentorship, telestration features for visual guidance during live procedures, and telepresence/telemonitoring, enabling remote proctoring and global collaboration [82–84]. These features contribute to more structured and scalable training pathways, potentially shortening the learning curve and enhancing procedural safety. Recognizing and addressing these learning curves through dedicated training and proctoring is paramount for ensuring the safe and effective adoption of MITS.

4.3. Barriers to widespread adoption

Despite the undeniable clinical advantages of MITS, several significant barriers impede their widespread adoption, particularly in resource-constrained environments. Addressing these challenges is crucial for ensuring equitable access to advanced surgical techniques globally.

One of the most prominent barriers is the cost of equipment and maintenance. Robotic surgical systems, in particular, represent a substantial capital investment, often costing millions of dollars in initial purchases. Beyond the upfront cost, there are ongoing expenses associated with disposable instruments, service contracts, and specialized operating room setups. These financial demands can be prohibitive for hospitals and healthcare systems, especially in developing countries, where budgets are often limited [33]. Although VATS is less expensive than RATS, the cost of HD video systems, specialized endoscopic instruments, and staplers can still be a significant barrier.

Access to technology is another critical challenge, particularly in regions with underdeveloped healthcare infrastructure. The distribution and availability of MITS equipment are often concentrated in urban centers and well-funded academic institutions, leaving rural and underserved areas with limited or no access to advanced surgical options. This creates disparities in care, where patients in certain geographical locations may not benefit from less invasive approaches due to a lack of local resources.

The steep learning curve for surgeons is a significant barrier to human intervention. As discussed, achieving proficiency in VATS and RATS requires dedicated training, extensive practice, and often mentorship. For busy surgeons in settings without structured training programs or access to experienced mentors, acquiring these skills can be challenging and time-consuming. The initial period of the learning curve may also be associated with longer operative times and potentially higher complication rates, which can deter surgeons and institutions from adopting these techniques [44].

Finally, reimbursement challenges can also hinder adoption. In some healthcare systems, the reimbursement rates for MITS procedures may not adequately cover the higher costs associated with specialized equipment and longer operative times, making it financially less attractive for hospitals to invest in and promote these techniques. Policy makers and healthcare payers need to recognize the long-term benefits of MITS, such as reduced hospital stays and fewer complications, which can lead to overall cost savings, and adjust reimbursement policies accordingly.

Overcoming these barriers requires a multi-faceted approach, including innovative financing models, the development of more affordable technologies, the expansion of accessible training programs, and supportive healthcare policies. Only through concerted efforts can the benefits of MITS be extended to a broader patient population worldwide.

4.4. Global trends in surgical volume and indications

Beyond mere adoption rates, analyzing global trends in surgical volume and the expanding indications for MITS provides a clearer picture of its evolving role. In many developed countries, MITS, particularly VATS, has become the preferred approach for early-stage lung cancer resections, including lobectomies and segmentectomies. This shift is driven by compelling evidence demonstrating equivalent oncological outcomes to open surgery, coupled with superior perioperative benefits [44]. The increasing global incidence of lung cancer, combined with advancements in screening and early detection, is further fueling the demand for minimally invasive approaches.

RATS is also experiencing a significant surge in volume, particularly for more complex procedures and in academic centers. Although initially adopted for mediastinal pathologies, RATS is increasingly being utilized for pulmonary resections, especially segmentectomies, where its enhanced dexterity and 3D visualization offer distinct advantages for precise anatomical dissection [17]. The continuous development of new robotic platforms and instruments is expected to further broaden its applications.

Beyond oncology, MITS is increasingly being utilized for a broader spectrum of benign intrathoracic and chest wall conditions [85]. Common indications now include pleural diseases, such as recurrent effusions and chylothorax, often managed via pleurodesis or thoracic duct ligation; mediastinal masses, such as thymectomy for myasthenia gravis; and chest wall deformities, including minimally invasive repair of pectus excavatum[86–90]. Additionally, MITS is being employed in selected cases of benign chest wall tumors and lesions, where reduced tissue trauma and improved cosmesis are particularly desirable. The benefits of reduced invasiveness, shorter hospitalization, and faster recovery are especially advantageous in benign conditions, where quality-of-life considerations often take precedence. This broadening of indications reflects growing surgical expertise, improved instrumentation, and a robust body of evidence supporting the safety and effectiveness of MITS across diverse thoracic pathologies.

However, it is important to note that the expansion of MITS is not without its challenges. The increasing complexity of cases being undertaken with minimally invasive procedures necessitates highly skilled surgical teams and robust perioperative support. Furthermore, the long-term outcomes of some newer MITS applications are still being studied, and ongoing research is crucial to ensure that the benefits outweigh any potential risks. Despite these considerations, the overarching trend is clear: MITS is becoming increasingly central to modern thoracic surgical practice, driven by its proven benefits and continuous technological evolution.

5. Future directions in minimally invasive thoracic surgery

The trajectory of MITS is a continuous innovation driven by technological convergence and a relentless pursuit of enhanced precision, safety, and patient outcomes. The coming decades are poised to witness transformative advancements, particularly with the integration of AI, AR, and the emergence of soft robotics, which promise to redefine the capabilities and accessibility of MITS.

5.1. Integration of artificial intelligence (AI)

AI is rapidly emerging as a powerful tool with the potential to revolutionize various aspects of thoracic surgery, from pre-operative planning to intraoperative guidance and post-operative care. AI algorithms, particularly those based on machine learning and deep learning (DL), can process vast amounts of data to identify patterns, make predictions, and assist in complex decision-making, thereby enhancing surgical precision and efficiency [91].

In surgical planning and navigation, AI can analyze patient-specific imaging data (CT, MRI, and PET scans) to create highly detailed 3D anatomical models. These models can be used to simulate surgical approaches, identify optimal resection planes, and predict potential challenges, allowing surgeons to meticulously plan complex procedures before entering the operating room. AI-powered navigation systems can then provide real-time guidance during surgery, overlaying critical anatomical structures and tumor boundaries onto the surgeon's view, thereby minimizing the risk of inadvertent injury to vital organs and ensuring complete tumor resection [92].

AI for image analysis and diagnosis holds immense promise in thoracic oncology. AI algorithms can be trained to detect subtle abnormalities in medical images, such as small lung nodules or early-stage cancers, with greater accuracy and speed than those of the human eye. This can lead to earlier diagnosis, which is crucial for improving patient prognosis. Furthermore, AI can assist in characterizing these lesions, differentiating between benign and malignant pathologies, and even predicting treatment response based on imaging biomarkers. Beyond diagnosis, AI can analyze pathological slides to assist in grading tumors and identifying molecular markers, guiding personalized treatment strategies.

Predictive analytics for patient outcomes represents a major application of AI in modern thoracic surgery and broader healthcare systems. By leveraging large datasets – including patient demographics, comorbidities, perioperative variables, and post-operative outcomes – AI models can stratify individual risk for complications, estimate length of stay, and even predict long-term survival trajectories. A range of predictive platforms has emerged to operationalize these insights. These systems extend beyond traditional health maintenance organizations to include integrated networks built on patient-centered care models. Notably, the University of California San Diego Health System has incorporated predictive algorithms directly into clinical workflows, using electronic health record (EHR) data combined with DL tools to facilitate early detection of critical conditions such as sepsis [93]. Another example is the PARAllel predictive MOdeling (PARAMO) platform, which employs EHR-driven analytics to optimize predictive modeling across patient cohorts. Its parallel-processing architecture significantly reduces computational time, enabling real-time risk stratification during high-demand clinical scenarios such as healthcare crises [93]. Collectively, these tools exemplify how AI-driven analytics can transform surgical decision-making, triage, and resource allocation by offering tailored, data-informed predictions for individual patients. This information can be invaluable for patient counseling, risk stratification, and optimizing perioperative management. For instance, AI could identify patients at high risk for post-operative pulmonary complications, allowing for targeted interventions to mitigate these risks. The integration of AI into MITS is expected to lead to more personalized, precise, and predictable surgical care, ultimately improving patient safety and outcomes.

5.2. Augmented reality (AR) and virtual reality (VR)

AR and VR technologies are poised to significantly enhance the capabilities of MITS, offering immersive visualization and interactive training platforms. While VR creates a completely simulated environment, AR overlays digital information onto the real world, providing surgeons with real-time, context-aware guidance during procedures [94].

AR for real-time surgical guidance is a particularly promising application. By projecting critical pre-operative imaging data (e.g., tumor location, vascular structures, airways) directly onto the patient during surgery, AR can provide surgeons with an "X-ray vision" capability. This allows for more precise tumor localization, safer dissection planes, and improved navigation in complex anatomical regions. For instance, an AR system could display the exact margins of a tumor or the course of a pulmonary artery directly on the patient's chest wall or within the endoscopic view, guiding the surgeon's movements with unprecedented accuracy. This real-time overlay of critical information can reduce operative time, minimize complications, and improve oncological outcomes, especially in challenging cases with atypical anatomy or small, non-palpable lesions [92].

VR for surgical training and simulation offers an immersive and highly realistic environment for surgeons to practice and refine their MITS skills without any risk to patients. VR simulators can replicate the visual and haptic feedback of actual surgical procedures, allowing trainees to repeatedly perform complex maneuvers, manage complications, and develop muscle memory. This is particularly valuable for mastering the intricacies of VATS and RATS, where hand-eye coordination and depth perception are crucial. VR training can also be used for pre-operative planning, allowing surgeons to virtually rehearse patient-specific surgeries, identify potential challenges, and optimize their approach before the actual procedure. The ability to practice in a controlled, repeatable environment can significantly shorten the learning curve, improve surgical proficiency, and enhance patient safety [95].

5.3. Soft robotics and miniaturization

The next frontier in minimally invasive surgery involves the development of soft robotics and further miniaturization of surgical instruments. Traditional rigid robotic instruments, while precise, can be limited in their ability to navigate tortuous anatomical pathways or conform to delicate tissue structures. Soft robots, made from compliant materials, offer inherent advantages in terms of flexibility, adaptability, and reduced risk of tissue damage, making them ideal for navigating complex and sensitive environments within the body [96].

Flexible and compliant robotic instruments are being designed to access previously unreachable areas within the thoracic cavity, such as small peripheral lung nodules or intricate bronchial tree segments. These robots can bend, twist, and change shape, allowing for safer navigation around vital structures and potentially enabling procedures that are currently too risky or technically challenging with rigid instruments. The inherent compliance of soft robots also means that they can interact with delicate tissues with less force, reducing the risk of perforation or injury. This is particularly relevant for procedures involving the lung parenchyma, which is highly susceptible to barotrauma or mechanical stress.

Furthermore, the drive toward smaller, more agile robotic systems aims to minimize the invasiveness of surgical access even further. This includes the development of microrobots that can be deployed through very small incisions or even natural orifices, potentially leading to incisionless surgery [97]. These miniaturized systems could enable highly localized interventions, reduce the systemic impact of surgery, and accelerate patient recovery. The ultimate goal is to create surgical robots that are not only precise but also highly adaptable and gentle, allowing for truly personalized and minimally disruptive interventions. The integration of soft robotics with advanced sensing capabilities and AI promises to unlock new possibilities for MITS, pushing the boundaries of what is surgically achievable with minimal patient impact [98].

5.4. Other emerging technologies

Beyond AI, AR/VR, and soft robotics, several other emerging technologies are poised to further enhance the capabilities of MITS, contributing to its ongoing evolution and refinement.

Enhanced visualization techniques continue to be the focus of innovation. This includes the development of multi-spectral imaging, which can provide information beyond the visible light spectrum, potentially revealing subtle physiological changes or tumor characteristics that are not visible to the naked eye. Confocal microscopy and optical coherence tomography (OCT) are also being explored for their potential to provide real-time, high-resolution imaging at the cellular level during surgery, allowing for immediate assessment of tissue pathology and surgical margins [5]. These advanced imaging modalities promise to provide surgeons with an even more detailed and informative view of the surgical field, leading to more precise resection and improved oncological outcomes.

Advanced energy sources are continually being refined to improve tissue dissection, hemostasis, and sealing. This includes innovations in ultrasonic, bipolar, and laser technologies, which aim for more efficient tissue cutting with minimal thermal spread, reduced smoke production, and improved safety profiles. The development of intelligent energy devices that can sense tissue impedance and automatically adjust energy delivery will further enhance their precision and reduce the risk of collateral damage [48].

Furthermore, the integration of intraoperative molecular imaging is gaining traction. This involves the use of fluorescent probes that specifically bind to cancer cells, making tumors glow during surgery. This real-time molecular guidance can help surgeons identify and remove all cancerous tissue, including microscopic foci that might otherwise be missed, thereby reducing recurrence rates and improving patient survival. This personalized approach to surgical oncology represents a significant step toward truly precision medicine in thoracic surgery.

Finally, the development of smart surgical instruments equipped with sensors and feedback mechanisms is ongoing. These instruments could provide real-time data on tissue tension, temperature, and even cellular characteristics, allowing surgeons to make more informed decisions during critical steps of the procedure. Such intelligent tools, combined with AI-driven analytics, could provide an unprecedented level of control and safety in MITS, further pushing the boundaries of what is achievable through minimally invasive approaches.

6. Conclusion

The evolution of MITS represents one of the most significant advancements in modern surgical practice, fundamentally transforming the approach to diseases of the chest. From the rudimentary thoracoscopic observations in the early twentieth century to the sophisticated robotic platforms and advanced imaging techniques of today, the journey of MITS has been characterized by relentless innovation and a steadfast commitment to improving patient care. The transition from open thoracotomy to VATS and subsequently to RATS has demonstrably reduced surgical invasiveness, leading to less post-operative pain, shorter hospital stays, faster recovery times, and improved cosmetic outcomes for a wide spectrum of thoracic pathologies.

Key technological advancements have been the driving force behind this evolution. HD and 3D imaging systems have provided surgeons with unparalleled visualization, while advanced endoscopic instrumentation, including energy devices and staplers, has enabled precise tissue manipulation and dissection through small incisions. The advent of robotic surgical systems has further increased the precision, dexterity, and ergonomic benefits for surgeons, making complex procedures more accessible and safer. These innovations have not only refined existing techniques but have also expanded the indications for MITS, allowing more patients to benefit from less invasive surgical interventions.

While the global adoption of MITS continues to grow, disparities persist, influenced by economic factors, healthcare infrastructure, and challenges associated with training and education. Overcoming these barriers requires concerted efforts to develop affordable technologies, establish robust training programs, and foster supportive healthcare policies. The learning curve for both VATS and RATS underscores the importance of structured curricula, simulation-based training, and mentorship to ensure surgeons' proficiency and patient safety.

The future of MITS is incredibly promising, with emerging technologies poised to usher in another era of transformative change. The integration of AI is set to revolutionize surgical planning, intraoperative navigation, and patient outcome prediction, leading to more personalized and precise care. AR will provide surgeons with real-time, context-aware guidance, enhancing accuracy and reducing complications. Furthermore, the development of soft robotics and continued miniaturization of instruments promises to enable even less invasive approaches, potentially leading to incisionless surgery and access to previously unreachable anatomical areas. These advancements, coupled with enhanced visualization techniques and smart surgical instruments, will continue to push the boundaries of what is surgically achievable with minimal patient impact.

In conclusion, MITS has redefined thoracic surgical practice, moving beyond mere technical innovations to fundamentally reshape patient experience and outcomes. As technology continues to advance and surgical expertise deepens, the evolution of MITS will undoubtedly continue, promising a future where surgical interventions are even safer, more precise, and profoundly less invasive, ultimately benefiting countless patients worldwide.

Author details

Ömer Faruk Sağlam
Thoracic Surgery, Tokat State Hospital, Tokat, Türkiye

*Address all correspondence to: mrfrksglm@gmail.com

References

[1] Jacobaeus HC. Über die Möglichkeit die Zystoskopie bei Untersuchung seröser Höhlungen anzuwenden. Münch Med Wochenschr. 1910;**57**:2090–2092.

[2] Hoksch B, Birken-Bertsch H, Müller JM. Thoracoscopy before Jacobaeus. The Annals of Thoracic Surgery. 2002;**74**:1288–1290. DOI: 10.1016/S0003-4975(02)03676-7.

[3] Sihoe ADL. The evolution of minimally invasive thoracic surgery: Implications for the practice of uniportal thoracoscopic surgery. J Thorac Disease. 2014;6:S604–17. doi:10.3978/j.issn.2072-1439.2014.08.52

[4] Bertolaccini L, Rocco G. History and development of minimally invasive surgery: VATS surgery. Shanghai Chest. 2019;**3**:16. DOI: 10.21037/shc.2019.03.01.

[5] Yutaka Y, Ng CSH. Editorial: Recent advances in minimally invasive thoracic surgery. Frontiers in Surgery. 2023; **10**:1182768. DOI: 10.3389/fsurg.2023.1182768.

[6] Wang L, Liu D, Lu J, Zhang S, Yang X. The feasibility and advantage of uniportal video-assisted thoracoscopic surgery (VATS) in pulmonary lobectomy. BMC Cancer. 2017;**17**:75. DOI: 10.1186/s12885-017-3069-z.

[7] Wang L, Ge L, Ren Y. Advantages and feasibility of intercostal nerve block in uniportal video-assisted thoracoscopic surgery (VATS). Postgraduate Medicine. 2023;**135**:472–479. DOI: 10.1080/00325481.2023.2187959.

[8] Bedetti B, Bertolaccini L, Solli P, Scarci M. Learning curve and established phase for uniportal VATS lobectomies: The Papworth experience. Journal of Thoracic Disease. 2017;**9**:138–142. DOI: 10.21037/jtd.2017.01.03.

[9] Wu N, Wu L, Qiu C, Yu Z, Xiang Y, Wang M, et al. A comparison of video-assisted thoracoscopic surgery with open thoracotomy for the management of chest trauma: A systematic review and meta-analysis. World Journal of Surgery. 2015;**39**:940–952

[10] Harris CG, James RS, Tian DH, Yan TD, Doyle MP, Gonzalez-Rivas D, et al. Systematic review and meta-analysis of uniportal versus multiportal video-assisted thoracoscopic lobectomy for lung cancer. Annals of Cardiothoracic Surgery. 2016;**5**:76–84

[11] Kakamad FH. Video-assisted thoracoscopic surgery (vats) versus thoracotomy in the treatment of pulmonary hydatid cysts: A randomized controlled trial. Health Science Reports. 2025;8. doi:10.1002/hsr2.70668

[12] Fung S, Jaber K, Kivilis M, Rehders A, Schauer A, Dizdar L, et al. Postoperative pain and clinical outcome following two- and three-port video-assisted thoracoscopic surgery for secondary spontaneous pneumothorax. Journal of Clinical Medicine. 2022;**11**:1404.

[13] Lim E, Batchelor TJP, Dunning J, Shackcloth M, Anikin V, Naidu B, et al. Video-assisted thoracoscopic or open lobectomy in early-stage lung cancer. NEJM Evidence. 2022:1. DOI: 10.1056/EVIDoa2100016.

[14] Zirafa CC, Romano G, Key TH, Davini F, Melfi F. The evolution of

robotic thoracic surgery. Annals of Cardiothoracic Surgery. 2019;**8**:210–217. DOI: 10.21037/acs.2019.03.03.

[15] Maraschi A, Fraccalini T, Bhakhri K. Robotic innovations in thoracic surgery: State of the art and future perspectives. surgical techniques and procedures [working title]. IntechOpen. 2025. doi:10.5772/intechopen.1009163

[16] Lazar JF, Hwalek AE. A review of robotic thoracic surgery adoption and future Innovations. Thoracic Surgery Clinics. 2023;**33**:1–10. DOI: 10.1016/j.thorsurg.2022.07.010.

[17] Tung KH, Yendamuri S, Seastedt KP. Adoption of the robotic platform across thoracic surgeries. Journal of Clinical Medicine. 2024;**13**:5764. DOI: 10.3390/jcm13195764.

[18] Sahai D, Nayak R. The evolution of vats and minimally invasive techniques in the treatment of lung cancer: A narrative review. Video-Assisted Thoracic Surgery. 2023;**8**:40–40. DOI: 10.21037/vats-22-63.

[19] Singer E, Kneuertz PJ, D'Souza DM, Moffatt-Bruce SD, Merritt RE. Understanding the financial cost of robotic lobectomy: Calculating the value of innovation? Annals of Cardiothoracic Surgery. 2019;**8**:194–201. DOI: 10.21037/acs.2018.05.18.

[20] Terra RM, Leite PHC, Dela Vega AJM. Global status of the robotic thoracic surgery. Journal of Thoracic Disease. 2021;**13**:6123–6128. DOI: 10.21037/jtd-19-3271.

[21] Yoshino I, Hashizume M, Shimada M, Tomikawa M, Tomiyasu M, Suemitsu R, et al. Thoracoscopic thymomectomy with the da Vinci computer-enhanced surgical system. The Journal of Thoracic and Cardiovascular Surgery. 2001;**122**: 783–785

[22] Lawrence L Adoption of VATS continues to vary globally - ILCN.org (ILCN/WCLC). IASLC Lung Cancer News 2021. https://www.ilcn.org/adoption-of-vats-continues-to-vary-globally/ (accessed June 26, 2025)

[23] Zhang J, Feng Q, Huang Y, Ouyang L, Luo F. Updated evaluation of robotic- and video-assisted thoracoscopic lobectomy or segmentectomy for lung cancer: A systematic review and meta-analysis. Frontiers in Oncology. 2022;12. DOI: 10.3389/fonc.2022.853530.

[24] Tosi D, Bottoni E, Palleschi A. Editorial: New perspectives in robotic-assisted thoracic surgery (RATS). Frontiers in Surgery. 2025;12. DOI: 10.3389/fsurg.2025.1574220.

[25] Gondé H, Laurent M, Gillibert A, Sarsam O-M, Varin R, Grimandi G, et al. The affordability of minimally invasive procedures in major lung resection: A prospective study. Interactive CardioVascular and Thoracic Surgery. 2017;**25**:469–475.

[26] Park SY, Suh JW, Narm KS, Lee CY, Lee JG, Paik HC, et al. Feasibility of four-arm robotic lobectomy as solo surgery in patients with clinical stage I lung cancer. Journal of Thoracic Disease. 2017;**9**:1607–1614.

[27] Zheng J, Wang Y, Zhang J, Guo W, Yang X, Luo L, et al. 5G ultra-remote robot-assisted laparoscopic surgery in China. Surgical Endoscopy. 2020;**34**:5172–5180.

[28] Enayati N, De Momi E, Ferrigno G. Haptics in robot-assisted surgery: Challenges and benefits. IEEE Reviews

in Biomedical Engineering. 2016;**9**: 49–65. DOI: 10.1109/RBME.2016. 2538080.

[29] Rae-Dupree J. Feel the precision: Next-gen robotic surgery with haptic feedback. IEEE Pulse. 2025;**16**:12–15. DOI: 10.1109/MPULS.2025.3526484.

[30] Gonzalez-Rivas D, Fieira E, Delgado M, Mendez L, Fernandez R, de la Torre M. Uniportal video-assisted thoracoscopic lobectomy. J Thorac Disease. 2013;**5** Suppl 3:S234-45. DOI: 10.3978/j.issn.2072-1439.2013.07.30.

[31] Melfi F. Early experience with robotic technology for thoracoscopic surgery. European Journal of Cardio-Thoracic Surgery. 2002;**21**: 864–868. DOI: 10.1016/S1010-7940(02)00102-1.

[32] Gonzalez-Rivas D, Bosinceanu M, Motas N, Manolache V. Uniportal robotic-assisted thoracic surgery for lung resections. European Journal of Cardio-Thoracic Surgery. 2022;62. doi:10.1093/ejcts/ezac410.

[33] Chen-Yoshikawa TF, Fukui T, Nakamura S, Ito T, Kadomatsu Y, Tsubouchi H, et al. Current trends in thoracic surgery. Nagoya Journal of Medical Science. 2020;**82**:161–174.

[34] Yotsukura M, Okubo Y, Yoshida Y, Nakagawa K, Watanabe S. Indocyanine green imaging for pulmonary segmentectomy. JTCVS Techniques. 2021;**6**:151–158. DOI: 10.1016/ j.xjtc.2020.12.005.

[35] Kim K, Jeon OH, Choi BH, Rho J, Lee JH, Eo JS, et al. Simultaneous visualization of lung tumor and intersegmental plane during pulmonary segmentectomy by intravenous injection of indocyanine green. Cancers (Basel). 2024;**16**:1439.

[36] Cui F, Liu J, Du M, Fan J, Fu J, Geng Q, et al. Expert consensus on indocyanine green fluorescence imaging for thoracoscopic lung resection (The version 2022). Translational Lung Cancer Research. 2022;**11**:2318–2331

[37] Olivera JA, Faith I, Onugha O. Novel uses of indocyanine green in thoracic surgery: A review and case series. Surgical Technology Online. 2023;43. DOI: 10.52198/23.STI.43. CV1706.

[38] Stasiak F, Seitlinger J, Streit A, Wollbrett C, Piccoli J, Siat J, et al. Sentinel lymph node in non-small cell lung cancer: assessment of feasibility and safety by near-infrared fluorescence imaging and clinical consequences. Journal of Personalized Medicine. 2022;**13**:90.

[39] Newton AD, Predina JD, Nie S, Low PS, Singhal S. Intraoperative fluorescence imaging in thoracic surgery. Journal of Surgical Oncology. 2018;**118**:344–355. DOI: 10.1002/ jso.25149.

[40] Géczi T, Simonka Z, Lantos J, Wetzel M, Szabó Z, Lázár G, et al. Near-infrared fluorescence guided surgery: State of the evidence from a health technology assessment perspective. Frontiers in Surgery. 2022:9. DOI: 10.3389/fsurg.2022.919739.

[41] Jiao Y, Liu Y, Jin M. Exploring the dark side of diagnostic dyes with a focus on Indocyanine green's adverse reactions. Scientific Reports. 2024; **14**:30155. DOI: 10.1038/s41598-024-81903-z.

[42] Thammineedi S. Visualisation of thoracic duct during esophagectomy by real-time fluorescent imaging—a technique in evolution. Diseases of the Esophagus. 2020;33. doi:10.1093/dote/doaa087.119.

[43] Morrell ALG, Morrell AC, Morrell-Junior AC, Mendes JM, Tustumi F, Morrell AG. Indocyanine green fluorescence imaging in robotic surgery: State of art, tips and tricks in current applications. Arquivos de Gastroenterologia. 2021;**58**:61–70. DOI: 10.1590/s0004-2803.202100000-11.

[44] Siu ICH, Li Z, CSH N. Latest technology in minimally invasive thoracic surgery. Annals of Translational Medicine. 2019;7:35–35. DOI: 10.21037/atm.2018.12.47.

[45] Sutton PA, Awad S, Perkins AC, Lobo DN. Comparison of lateral thermal spread using monopolar and bipolar diathermy, the Harmonic Scalpel™ and the Ligasure™. British Journal of Surgery. 2010;**97**:428–433. DOI: 10.1002/bjs.6901.

[46] Gabryel P, Kasprzyk M, Roszak M, Campisi A, Smoliński S, Zieliński P, et al. Comparison of the LigaSure™ bipolar vessel sealer to monopolar electrocoagulation for thoracoscopic lobectomy and lymphadenectomy: A prospective randomized controlled trial. Surgical Endoscopy. 2023;**37**:4449–4457

[47] Milsom JW, Trencheva K, Momose K, Peev MP, Christos P, Shukla PJ, et al. A pilot randomized controlled trial comparing THUNDERBEAT to the Maryland LigaSure energy device in laparoscopic left colon surgery. Surgical Endoscopy. 2022;**36**:4265–4274

[48] Bertolaccini L, Pardolesi A, Solli P. Technological advancements in thoracic surgery: A brief introduction to the future. Journal of Visualized Surgery. 2017;**3**:37. DOI: 10.21037/jovs.2017.02.08.

[49] Miller DL, Roy S, Kassis ES, Yadalam S, Ramisetti S, Johnston SS. Impact of powered and tissue-specific endoscopic stapling technology on clinical and economic outcomes of video-assisted thoracic surgery lobectomy procedures: A retrospective, observational study. Advances in Therapy. 2018;**35**:707–723. DOI: 10.1007/s12325-018-0679-z.

[50] Tsunezuka Y, Tanaka N, Fujimori H. The impact of endoscopic stapler selection on bleeding at the vascular stump in pulmonary artery transection. medical devices. Evidence and Research. 2020;**13**:41–47. DOI: 10.2147/MDER.S240343.

[51] Cao Y, Xiong F, Xia X, Gu P, Wang Q, Wu A, et al. Economic impact of powered stapler in video-assisted thoracic surgery lobectomy for lung cancer in a Chinese tertiary hospital: A cost-minimization analysis. Health Economics Review. 2022;**12**:12

[52] Redmann JG, Lavin TE, French MS, Broussard TD, Lapointe-Gagner M. Improving Hemostasis in Sleeve Gastrectomy With Alternative Stapler. Journal of the Society of Laparoscopic & Robotic Surgeons. 2020;**24**: e2020.00073. doi:10.4293/JSLS.2020.00073

[53] Wottawa CR, Genovese B, Nowroozi BN, Hart SD, Bisley JW, Grundfest WS, et al. Evaluating tactile feedback in robotic surgery for potential clinical application using an animal model. Surgical Endoscopy. 2016;**30**:3198–3209.

[54] Abeywardena S, Yuan Q, Tzemanaki A, Psomopoulou E, Droukas L, Melhuish C, et al. Estimation of tool-tissue forces in robot-assisted minimally invasive surgery using neural networks. Frontiers in Robotics and AI. 2019:6. DOI: 10.3389/frobt.2019.00056.

[55] Alleblas CCJ, Vleugels MPH, Stommel MWJ, Nieboer TE. Performance of a haptic feedback grasper in laparoscopic surgery: a randomized pilot comparison with conventional graspers in a porcine model. Surgical Innovation. 2019;**26**:573–580. DOI: 10.1177/1553350619848551.

[56] Gamal A, Moschovas MC, Saikali S, Reddy S, Ozawa Y, Sharma R, et al. Comparing the technological and intraoperative performances of da vinci xi and davinci 5 robotic platforms in patients undergoing robotic-assisted radical prostatectomy. International Brazilian Journal of Urology. 2025:51. DOI: 10.1590/s1677-5538.ibju.2024.0569.

[57] Pacchierotti C, Prattichizzo D, Kuchenbecker KJ. cutaneous feedback of fingertip deformation and vibration for palpation in robotic surgery. IEEE Transactions on Biomedical Engineering. 2016;**63**:278–287. DOI: 10.1109/TBME.2015.2455932.

[58] Wei S, Chen M, Chen N, Liu L. Feasibility and safety of robot-assisted thoracic surgery for lung lobectomy in patients with non-small cell lung cancer: A systematic review and meta-analysis. World Journal of Surgical Oncology. 2017;**15**:98. DOI: 10.1186/s12957-017-1168-6.

[59] Salkowski M, Checcucci E, Chow AK, Rogers CC, Adbollah F, Liatsikos E, et al. New multiport robotic surgical systems: A comprehensive literature review of clinical outcomes in urology. Therapeutic Advances in Urology. 2023:15. DOI: 10.1177/17562872231177781.

[60] Othman W, Lai Z-HA, Abril C, Barajas-Gamboa JS, Corcelles R, Kroh M, et al. Tactile sensing for minimally invasive surgery: Conventional methods and potential emerging tactile technologies. Front Robot AI. 2022:8. DOI: 10.3389/frobt.2021.705662.

[61] Kohjimoto Y, Yamashita S, Iwagami S, Muraoka S, Wakamiya T, Hara I. Hinotori™ vs. da Vinci®: Propensity score-matched analysis of surgical outcomes of robot-assisted radical prostatectomy. Journal of Robotic Surgery. 2024;**18**:130. DOI: 10.1007/s11701-024-01877-y.

[62] Yu DY, Chang YW, Lee HY, Kim WY, Kim HY, Lee JB, et al. Detailed comparison of the da Vinci Xi and S surgical systems for transaxillary thyroidectomy. Medicine. 2021:100: e24370. DOI: 10.1097/MD.0000000000024370.

[63] Lee J, Hong DG. Comparative study of supracervical hysterectomy between da Vinci SP® surgical system and conventional single-site laparoscopy for uterine fibroid: Single center experiences. Journal of Robotic Surgery. 2023;**17**:1421–1427. DOI: 10.1007/s11701-023-01527-9.

[64] Matsuura M, Nagao S, Kurokawa S, Tamate M, Akimoto T, Saito T. Surgical outcomes of da Vinci Xi™ and da Vinci SP™ for early-stage endometrial cancer in patients undergoing hysterectomy. Journal of Clinical Medicine. 2024;**13**:2864. DOI: 10.3390/jcm13102864.

[65] Miyamura H, Takada K, Ohwaki A, Kobayashi A, Ito M, Nomura H, et al.

Initial experience and surgical outcomes of robotic-assisted total hysterectomy using the da Vinci SPTM surgical system. Asian Journal of Endoscopic Surgery. 2024:17. DOI: 10.1111/ases.13298.

[66] Seon KE, Lee YJ, Lee J-Y, Nam EJ, Kim S, Kim YT, et al. Comparing surgical outcomes of da Vinci SP and da Vinci Xi for endometrial cancer surgical staging in a propensity score-matched study. Scientific Reports. 2023;**13**:11752. DOI: 10.1038/s41598-023-37659-z.

[67] Jiahai C, You L, Jianping G, Yakun W. Application of da Vinci surgical robotic system in hepatobiliary surgery. International Journal of Surgery and Medicine. 2017;1. DOI: 10.5455/ijsm.da-Vinci-surgical-robotic-system-in-hepatobiliary-surgery.

[68] Chan JWY, PSY Y, Yang JH, Yuan EQ, Jia H, Peng J, et al. Surgical access trauma following minimally invasive thoracic surgery. European Journal of Cardio-Thoracic Surgery. 2020;**58**: i6–13

[69] Bendixen M, Jørgensen OD, Kronborg C, Andersen C, Licht PB. Postoperative pain and quality of life after lobectomy via video-assisted thoracoscopic surgery or anterolateral thoracotomy for early stage lung cancer: A randomised controlled trial. The Lancet Oncology. 2016;**17**:836–844. DOI: 10.1016/S1470-2045(16)00173-X.

[70] Oda R, Okuda K, Osaga S, Watanabe T, Sakane T, Tatematsu T, et al. Long-term outcomes of video-assisted thoracoscopic surgery lobectomy vs. thoracotomy lobectomy for stage IA non-small cell lung cancer. Surgery Today. 2019;**49**:369–377

[71] Veronesi G, Novellis P, Voulaz E, Alloisio M. Robot-assisted surgery for lung cancer: State of the art and perspectives. Lung Cancer: Targets and Therapy. 2016;**101**:28–34. DOI: 10.1016/j.lungcan.2016.09.004.

[72] Paladini P, Meniconi F, Ghisalberti M, Luzzi L, Ligabue T, De LL, et al. Review of the learning curve of video-assisted thoracic surgery & robotic-assisted thoracic surgery lobectomies—similarities and differences. Current Challenges in Thoracic Surgery. 2021;**3**:16–16

[73] Huang S, Huang X, Huang Z, Luo R, Liang W. Comparison of robot-assisted thoracic surgery versus video-assisted thoracic surgery in the treatment of lung cancer: A systematic review and meta-analysis of prospective studies. Frontiers in Oncology. 2023;13. doi:10.3389/fonc.2023.1271709

[74] Habibi Nameghi F, Oghogho A, Baltag D, Szafron B, Viola C, Kadlec J, et al. Outcomes of RATS in comparison to VATS and open lung resections for malignancy in propensity matched high-risk patients. Journal of Robotic Surgery. 2025;**19**:225.

[75] Harrison OJ, Maraschi A, Routledge T, Lampridis S, LeReun C, Bille A. A cost analysis of robotic vs. video-assisted thoracic surgery: The impact of the learning curve and the COVID-19 pandemic. Frontiers in Surgery. 2023;**10**. DOI: 10.3389/fsurg.2023.1123329.

[76] Wilson-Smith AR, Anning N, Muston B, Eranki A, Williams ML, Wilson-Smith CJ, et al. The learning curve of the robotic-assisted lobectomy

—a systematic review and meta-analysis. Annals of Cardiothoracic Surgery. 2023;**12**:1–8.

[77] Potter AL, Spasojevic A, Raman V, Hurd JC, Senthil P, Mathey-Andrews C, et al. The increasing adoption of minimally invasive lobectomy in the United States. The Annals of Thoracic Surgery. 2023;**116**:222–229.

[78] Re Cecconi E, Mangiameli G, De Simone M, Cioffi U, Marulli G, Testori A. Vats lobectomy for lung cancer. What has been the evolution over the time? Frontiers in Oncology. 2024;13. DOI: 10.3389/fonc.2023.1268362.

[79] Kaur MN, Xie F, Shiwcharan A, Patterson L, Shargall Y, Finley C, et al. Robotic versus video-assisted thoracoscopic lung resection during early program development. The Annals of Thoracic Surgery. 2018;**105**:1050–1057

[80] Kim SS, Schumacher L, Cooke DT, Servais E, Rice D, Sarkaria I, et al. The society of thoracic surgeons expert consensus statements on a framework for a standardized national robotic curriculum for thoracic surgery trainees. The Annals of Thoracic Surgery. 2025;**119**:719–732

[81] Massard G, Tabin N, Konge L, Frick AE, Batirel H, Brunelli A, et al. Training curriculum for European thoracic surgeons: A joint initiative of the European Society of Thoracic Surgeons and the European Respiratory Society. European Journal of Cardio-Thoracic Surgery. 2020;**57**:418–421.

[82] Cristofari H, Jung MK, Niclauss N, Toso C, Kloetzer L. Teaching and learning robotic surgery at the dual console: A video-based qualitative analysis. Journal of Robotic Surgery. 2022;**16**:169–178. DOI: 10.1007/s11701-021-01224-5.

[83] Castaldi MT, Palmer M, Con J, Bergamaschi R. Robotic-assisted surgery training (RAST): Assessment of surgeon console ergonomic skills. Journal of Surgical Education. 2023;**80**:1723–1735. DOI: 10.1016/j.jsurg.2023.08.019.

[84] Rahimi AM, Uluç E, Hardon SF, Bonjer HJ, van der Peet Dl, Daams F. Training in robotic-assisted surgery: A systematic review of training modalities and objective and subjective assessment methods. Surgical Endoscopy. 2024;**38**:3547–3555. DOI: 10.1007/s00464-024-10915-7.

[85] Minervini F, Sergi CM, Scarci M, Kestenholz PB, Valentini L, Boschetti L, et al. Benign tumors of the chest wall. Journal of Thoracic Disease. 2024;**16**:722–736.

[86] Fahimi H, Casselman FP, Mariani MA, van Boven Wj, Knaepen PJ, van Swieten HA. Current management of postoperative chylothorax. The Annals of Thoracic Surgery. 2001;**71**:448–450. DOI: 10.1016/S0003-4975(00)02033-6.

[87] Perikleous P, Rathinam S, Waller DA. VATS and open chest surgery in diagnosis and treatment of benign pleural diseases. Journal of Visualized Surgery. 2017;**3**:84–84. DOI: 10.21037/jovs.2017.05.03.

[88] Sundaralingam A, Grabczak EM, Burra P, Costa MI, George V, Harriss E, et al. ERS statement on benign pleural effusions in adults. European Respiratory Journal. 2024;**64**: 2302307. 2302307. DOI: 10.1183/13993003.02307-2023.

[89] Nuss D, Obermeyer RJ, Kelly RE. Nuss bar procedure: Past, present and future. Annals of Cardiothoracic Surgery. 2016;**5**:422–433. DOI: 10.21037/acs.2016.08.05.

[90] Bagheri R, Boonstani R, Sadrizadeh A, Salehi M, Afghani R, Rahnama A, et al. Thymectomy for nonthymomatous myasthenia gravis. Innovations: Technology and Techniques in Cardiothoracic and Vascular Surgery. 2018;**13**:77–80.

[91] Leivaditis V, Maniatopoulos AA, Lausberg H, Mulita F, Papatriantafyllou A, Liolis E, et al. Artificial intelligence in thoracic surgery: A review bridging innovation and clinical practice for the next generation of surgical care. Journal of Clinical Medicine. 2025;**14**:2729.

[92] Sadeghi AH, Mank Q, Tuzcu AS, Hofman J, Siregar S, Maat A, et al. Artificial intelligence–assisted augmented reality robotic lung surgery: Navigating the future of thoracic surgery. JTCVS Techniques. 2024;**26**:121–125.

[93] Boukenze B Disease forecasting and patient monitoring: The great role of medical data analytics. 2023 International Conference on Networking, Sensing and Control (ICNSC), IEEE; 2023, p. 1–6. DOI: 10.1109/ICNSC58704.2023.10319039.

[94] Doornbos M-CJ, Peek JJ, Maat APWM, Ruurda JP, de Backer P, Cornelissen BMW, et al. Augmented reality implementation in minimally invasive surgery for future application in pulmonary surgery: A systematic review. Surgical Innovation. 2024;**31**:646–658

[95] Dagnino G, Kundrat D. Robot-assistive minimally invasive surgery: Trends and future directions. International Journal of Intelligent Robotics and Applications. 2024;**8**:812–826. DOI: 10.1007/s41315-024-00341-2.

[96] Runciman M, Darzi A, Mylonas GP. Soft robotics in minimally invasive surgery. Soft Robotics. 2019;**6**:423–443. DOI: 10.1089/soro.2018.0136.

[97] Dolph E, Krause C, Oleynikov D. Future Robotic Systems: Microrobotics and Autonomous Robots. Robotic-Assisted Minimally Invasive Surgery. Cham: Springer International Publishing; 2019. pp. 329–335. DOI: 10.1007/978-3-319-96866-7_40.

[98] Zhu J, Lyu L, Xu Y, Liang H, Zhang X, Ding H, et al. Intelligent soft surgical robots for next-generation minimally invasive surgery. Advanced Intelligent Systems. 2021:3. DOI: 10.1002/aisy.202100011.

Chapter 5

Robotic Subxiphoid Thymectomy: Approaches and Techniques

Padungkiat Tangpiroontham and Krit Vikan

Abstract

Robotic subxiphoid thymectomy presents a minimally invasive surgical approach that provides comparable visualization of the operative field to that achieved during a median sternotomy. This technique facilitates the effective exposure of critical anatomical structures, including the bilateral phrenic nerves and significant cervical structures, such as the innominate vein. The initial method was described as involving direct subxiphoid dissection followed by the placement of bilateral intercostal space ports. Subsequently, several variations have been developed, including the single-port approach utilizing the da Vinci SP (single port) system and the double-docking technique proposed by Tangpiroontham. In this article, the authors provide a comprehensive overview of the various robotic subxiphoid thymectomy techniques, emphasizing their respective advantages and limitations in terms of the extent of subxiphoid muscular dissection, the number and configuration of port placements, and other pertinent surgical considerations.

Keywords: robotic thymectomy, subxiphoid thymectomy, uniportal subxiphoid thymectomy, multiportal subxiphoid thymectomy, Tangpiroontham, Chao, Suda

1. Introduction

Thymectomy remains a cornerstone in the treatment of thymic epithelial tumors (TET) and myasthenia gravis (MG), aiming for complete removal of the thymus and perithymic fat to optimize oncologic and functional outcomes. Historically, the median sternotomy was the gold standard, providing excellent exposure to the anterior mediastinum, both phrenic nerves, and cervical thymic extensions. Although effective in achieving complete resection, this approach was associated with significant drawbacks, including extensive tissue trauma, postoperative pain, risk of sternal wound complications, and prominent scarring.

To reduce morbidity, the transcervical thymectomy was introduced in the 1980s as a less invasive option. Through a collar incision in the lower neck, surgeons could resect the thymus without dividing the sternum. This approach offered superior cosmetic results and shorter recovery times, but its limitations included restricted visualization of the inferior poles and pericardial fat, as well as technical challenges in achieving complete clearance, particularly in oncologic cases.

In the 1990s, video-assisted thoracoscopic surgery (VATS) thymectomy emerged as a minimally invasive alternative. By using small intercostal ports and thoracoscopic visualization, VATS thymectomy offered reduced postoperative pain, shorter hospitalization, faster recovery, and improved cosmetic outcomes compared with sternotomy. However, its limitations – two-dimensional imaging, constrained instrument articulation, and difficulty accessing the contralateral hemithorax – restricted its effectiveness in some cases, especially those requiring complete bilateral dissection.

The introduction of robotic-assisted thoracic surgery (RATS) marked a paradigm shift. Robotic platforms, such as the da Vinci system, offer three-dimensional (3D) high-definition vision, tremor elimination, and articulated instruments with seven degrees of freedom, greatly enhancing precision and safety in dissection around vital structures. Within RATS, several approaches have been developed, including the lateral transthoracic approach, bilateral intercostal approach, and subcostal approach. These methods allow excellent exposure for many anterior mediastinal resections, with each having distinct advantages and drawbacks in terms of visualization, ergonomics, and ease of specimen retrieval. However, limitations remain – particularly in consistently visualizing both phrenic nerves and the upper poles of the thymus in a single field – leading to continued refinement of access strategies.

The robotic subxiphoid thymectomy (RST) utilizes a subxiphoid entry – via multiportal or uniportal configurations. This technique provides a central, symmetrical view of the anterior mediastinum and consistent visualization of both phrenic nerves without sternal division. This approach facilitates *en bloc* removal of the thymus and surrounding mediastinal fat with minimal intercostal nerve trauma, potentially lowering postoperative pain and accelerating recovery. RST is also adaptable to complex resections, reoperations, and extended thymectomies, often improving surgeon ergonomics.

This chapter explores RST in detail, encompassing multiportal and uniportal approaches, and provides a comparative analysis with other robotic thymectomy techniques. Innovative adaptations, such as the double-docking technique, and unique institutional protocols are also discussed. Other robotic thymectomy techniques beyond the subxiphoid approach are not covered in depth in this chapter.

2. Techniques in robotic thymectomy

RATS for thymectomy has evolved with multiple approaches, including lateral (right and left) transthoracic and subxiphoid. The robotic platform allows greater freedom of movement, improved 3D visualization, and fine dissection capabilities. The use of CO_2 insufflation creates a working space in the mediastinum, allowing the surgeon to mobilize the thymus and pericardial fat en bloc [1]. Although lateral approaches have been historically preferred, limitations include restricted visualization and exposure of the contralateral phrenic nerve, innominate vein, and difficulty accessing both hemithoraces for extended thymectomy. Moreover, it is associated with intercostal nerve pain postoperatively. Consequently, the subxiphoid approach has gained traction.

2.1 Subxiphoid thymectomy

The subxiphoid approach offers a central vantage point with bilateral mediastinal exposure, providing ideal visualization for total and extended thymectomy, particularly in MG patients. Subxiphoid access avoids intercostal nerve trauma and permits easy identification of both phrenic nerves, which are crucial structures to be identified during the operation. The technique can be performed using multiportal or uniportal robotic configurations.

2.1.1 Multiportal subxiphoid approach: Suda's technique

This approach was developed by Suda T. After general anesthesia and patient positioning in the supine position with legs apart and slight reverse Trendelenburg, differential pulmonary ventilation may not be required. Positive-end expiratory pressure is not used in order to prevent the lungs from protruding during surgery and interfering with the procedure. A 3-cm horizontal or vertical skin incision is made 1 cm inferior to the xiphoid process. The xiphoid is separated from the rectus abdominis to facilitate entry into the retrosternal space. Blunt finger dissection is used to develop the preperitoneal plane. The GelPOINT Mini, fitted with two child ports, is inserted to maintain the subxiphoid access. CO_2 is insufflated at 8 mmHg to enlarge the anterior mediastinal space. A rigid endoscope with a 5-mm diameter (30° perspective) and the LigaSure Maryland Jaw (Covidien, Mansfield, MA) are used to separate the thymus gland from the posterior aspect of the sternum. Both pleural cavities are opened. Da Vinci surgical ports (8 mm) are then inserted under thoracoscopic guidance, one in each hemithorax through the sixth intercostal space, anterior axillary line. The da Vinci robotic system (commonly Si or Xi) is docked centrally. The 30° camera is inserted through the subxiphoid port. A monopolar spatula or bipolar Maryland forceps is attached to the right-arm, and either bipolar fenestrated grasping forceps or Cadiere forceps is attached to the left arm. The EndoWrist Vessel Sealer (Intuitive Surgical) may be used, which allows safe sealing and separation of vessels. Another GelPOINT Mini port is introduced with Autonomy Grasper 45-cm forceps (Cambridge Endo), used by the surgical assistant.

The dissection begins caudally along the pericardium and progresses cranially toward the innominate vein. Both phrenic nerves are visualized and preserved throughout. The upper poles of the thymus are dissected from the thyrothymic ligament. The thymic veins are dissected using the EndoWrist Vessel Sealer. The entire thymus, along with surrounding fat, is removed *en bloc*. The specimen is retrieved inside a bag via the subxiphoid port, and hemostasis is confirmed. A 20-Fr chest tube is placed through one of the subcostal ports, and the subxiphoid wound is closed in layers. Suda et al. reported favorable operative times and reduced blood loss using this method [2].

2.1.2 Multiportal subxiphoid approach: Chao's technique

Chao's operative steps involve placing the patient in the supine position with both arms abducted to allow unobstructed access [3]. The operative table is adjusted to a slight reverse Trendelenburg position. General anesthesia with single-lumen endotracheal tube intubation is performed. A vertical midline incision (approximately 3–4 cm) is created just below the xiphoid process. The xiphoid process is resected to create a working channel into the retrosternal space. Blunt dissection is performed blindly to create a preperitoneal and retrosternal pocket. Then, a 2- to 3-cm longitudinal incision is made on the rectus abdominis fascia. An extra-small wound retractor (with a 6½ surgical glove placed on its outer ring) is inserted into this subxiphoid wound. Two trocars are positioned upon removal of two glove fingers. A thoracoscopic camera and a LigaSure device are securely introduced into the chest. CO_2 is insufflated at 8 mmHg to expand the anterior mediastinal space. A deeper dissection between the lower retrosternum and the anterior mediastinum is performed using LigaSure. Under thoracoscopic guidance, bilateral 1-cm working ports (for two 8-mm trocars) are placed in the sixth intercostal space along the anterior axillary lines. The da Vinci Xi robotic system is then docked from the patient's left side. A 30° camera is introduced via the subxiphoid port, with ProGrasp forceps and the monopolar curved scissors attached to the left and right arms, respectively.

The dissection starts from the right lower pole of the thymus, at the pericardiophrenic angle, and then proceeds to the left lower pole. Subsequently, the operation continues to the thymic upper pole. Special attention is given to preserving both phrenic nerves, which are fully visualized due to the midline approach. The right and left upper thymic poles are resected caudally toward the innominate vein. Downward traction on the thymus is adequately applied during these procedures. Thymic vessels are sealed with Hem-o-lok clips. Near-infrared fluorescence imaging is applied during surgery. The pericardiophrenic neurovascular bundle is clearly visible using an Indocyanine green (ICG) injection. The specimen is removed through the subxiphoid port. A chest tube is not routinely used.

2.1.3 Uniportal subxiphoid approach

Suda et al. [2] also pioneered a true uniportal RST using a single subxiphoid incision with a multichannel access port. The patient is placed in the supine position, and a vertical 3–4 cm incision is made just below the xiphoid process. The xiphoid process is excised to allow entrance into the retrosternal space. A glove port or commercial single-access port (e.g., GelPOINT) is inserted through the incision. CO_2 is insufflated at 6–10 mmHg to expand the anterior mediastinum. The da Vinci Si system is used, and all robotic instruments, including the 30° camera and working instruments (e.g., Maryland bipolar forceps, monopolar scissors), are inserted through the single multichannel port. Dissection begins at the caudal edge of the thymus and proceeds cranially. The anterior mediastinal fat and thymic tissue are dissected from the pericardium and great vessels. Both phrenic nerves are clearly visualized. Thymic veins are clipped or sealed near the innominate vein. The superior poles are dissected free from the thyrothymic ligaments, and the specimen is extracted through the same subxiphoid port.

Although technically demanding due to instrument crowding and reduced triangulation, this technique offers excellent cosmetic outcomes, reduced intercostal nerve trauma, and suitable access for early-stage thymic tumors or in MG. This uniportal robotic subxiphoid approach represents the most minimally invasive option currently available for thymectomy. Early series report equivalent oncologic safety, shorter operative time, and a lower conversion rate to multi-port surgery with growing institutional experience [2].

2.1.4 Uniportal subxiphoid approach, using da Vinci SP

The uniportal RST using the da Vinci SP (single port) system was initially proposed by Chao. It represents a technological innovation that merges robotic dexterity with the cosmetic and ergonomic benefits of a single-incision technique. The system utilizes a single 2.5 cm cannula to introduce a 3D flexible camera and three articulating robotic instruments. These instruments offer maneuverability in confined anatomical spaces while minimizing the risk of instrument clashing.

This approach begins with the patient in the open-legged supine position, with both arms abducted. Routine ventilation is performed using two-lung ventilation with reduced tidal volumes; however, one-lung ventilation is selectively utilized in cases where tumors invade adjacent structures. A vertical 2.5–4 cm incision is created 1–2 cm below the xiphoid process. The skin and subcutaneous tissues are dissected, taking care not to damage the peritoneum. Blunt finger dissection is performed to create space between the preperitoneal and retrosternal areas. A multichannel access platform, such as Lapsingle Vision (Sejong Medical, Gyeonggi, Republic of Korea) or SP Access Port (Intuitive Surgical Inc.), is inserted into the subxiphoid wound. CO_2 insufflation at 6–10 mmHg expands the anterior mediastinal space.

The floating dock technique is necessary in this approach. The cannula tip is docked onto the tip of the multi-channel port and floated above the incision. The port of entry floats above the incision. The da Vinci cart is docked from the right side, and a robotic scope is introduced into the lower middle hole. Fenestrated bipolar forceps, Cadiere forceps, and a monopolar scissor were utilized as per the surgeon's preference. Dissection is performed. The bilateral mediastinal pleura are opened after dissection of the tissues beneath the xiphoid process. Then, the robotic scope is repositioned at the upper middle hole, and the Cadiere forceps are added at the lower middle hole. The procedure is carried out similarly to the conventional subxiphoid RATS thymectomy. After the specimen is retrieved, two chest drains (Evacuator Barovac, 100 mL, Sewoon Medical Co., Seoul, Republic of Korea) are inserted into the bilateral pleural cavity through a subxiphoid incision.

This technique eliminates intercostal incisions, allows clear exposure of both phrenic nerves, and important structures. The articulating instruments of the SP system also enhance dissection precision. However, this approach requires specialized SP robotic systems, limits assistant access through separate ports, and involves a steep learning curve due to the complexity of instrument coordination. Early experience has shown comparable oncologic outcomes with the potential benefits of improved cosmesis, reduced postoperative discomfort, and a shorter hospital stay [4]. Data reported by Lee JH et al. [5] have demonstrated a lower conversion rate to multi-port surgery, shorter chest tube drainage duration, and a shorter postoperative hospital stay compared to subxiphoid single-port VATS.

2.1.5 Subxiphoid approach, double-docking technique

Although conventional RATS subxiphoid thymectomy techniques provide excellent visualization, they require a 3–4 cm vertical subxiphoid incision, which may lead to inferior cosmetic outcomes, risk of injury to branches of the musculophrenic artery, unintentional peritoneal entry, damage to the rectus abdominis muscle, and necessitate specialized port devices.

To address these limitations, the double-docking technique, proposed by Tangpiroontham, introduces two separate robotic docking phases. This approach enhances visualization of the major vascular structures and both phrenic nerves, improves instrument maneuverability, and reduces external robotic arm collisions, resulting in a more ergonomic and effective surgical workflow. In addition, this approach is beneficial in centers without integrated table motion with the da Vinci system.

Initial port placement side depends on the side of the tumor. In MG patients, a left-sided approach is preferred to facilitate complete clearance of the thymus gland from the left phrenic nerve. The patient is placed in a semi-lateral position. The operative side is elevated, the ipsilateral arm is fixed at a lower position than the bed, and the contralateral arm is placed in an abducted position. General anesthesia is administered via a double-lumen endotracheal tube. The procedure begins with subxiphoid dissection performed using a two-port RATS setup, unlike conventional techniques whereby no subxiphoid VATS dissection is required, then transitioning to a three-port RATS configuration. CO_2 is insufflated at 6–12 mmHg. Initially, only the camera and a da Vinci Vessel Sealer Extend or curved-tip dissector are used.

The approach described here is tailored for left-sided access, as demonstrated in an attached video; for thymic tumors predominantly located on the right, the setup is reversed accordingly. A thoracoscope is introduced through the left eighth intercostal space at the anterior axillary line, with an additional working port in the left sixth intercostal space at the midaxillary line (see **Figure 1a**). A Vessel Sealer Extend facilitates dissection around the subxiphoid area, beginning at the mediastinal pleura and extending caudally to the diaphragm. After diaphragm exposure, the dissection progresses into the mediastinal pleura in the mid-chest area, then enters the right pleural cavity. Once the right pleural cavity is entered, the dissection is performed further at the subxiphoid area. The branch of the musculophrenic artery is controlled with a Vessel Sealer Extend. An 8-mm subxiphoid incision, just below the xiphoid process, is then created. A clamp is inserted to access the cavity, allowing subsequent placement of an 8-mm robotic port. Upon entry, the Vessel Sealer Extend may also be used to gently depress the heart during this maneuver (see **Figure 2a**). A fenestrated bipolar dissector is introduced through this subxiphoid port to initiate thymectomy on the left side. Dissection closely follows, but care is taken not to injure the left phrenic nerve to ensure complete thymic removal. Superior dissection continues along the mediastinal pleura to expose the upper sternum. An additional 8-mm port is placed into the right pleural cavity under direct vision, mirroring the left side (see **Figure 2b**). At this point, the da Vinci Vessel Sealer Extend is undocked and redocked through the subxiphoid position. The operating table is subsequently adjusted to turn the patient to a supine orientation. This configuration (thoracoscopic at the subxiphoid incision, fenestrated bipolar dissector at the patient's right-sided robotic port, and a Vessel Sealer Extend at the patient's left-side robotic port) offers exceptional visualization of the anterior mediastinum and both phrenic nerves, nearly similar to an open sternotomy (see **Figure 2c**). The prior thoracoscopic port at the left eighth intercostal space is currently utilized as an assistant port (see **Figure 1b**). Dissection continues to clear thymic tissue from the sternum and mediastinal pleura, proceeding toward the right phrenic nerve. The right thymic lobe is

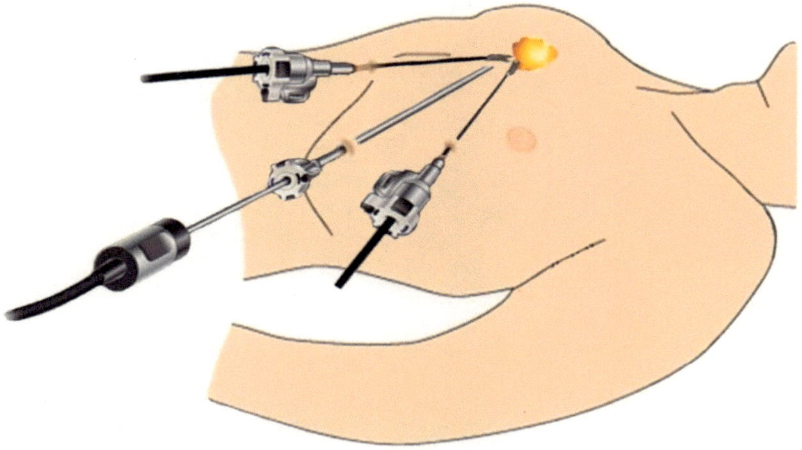

(a) First, lateral docking

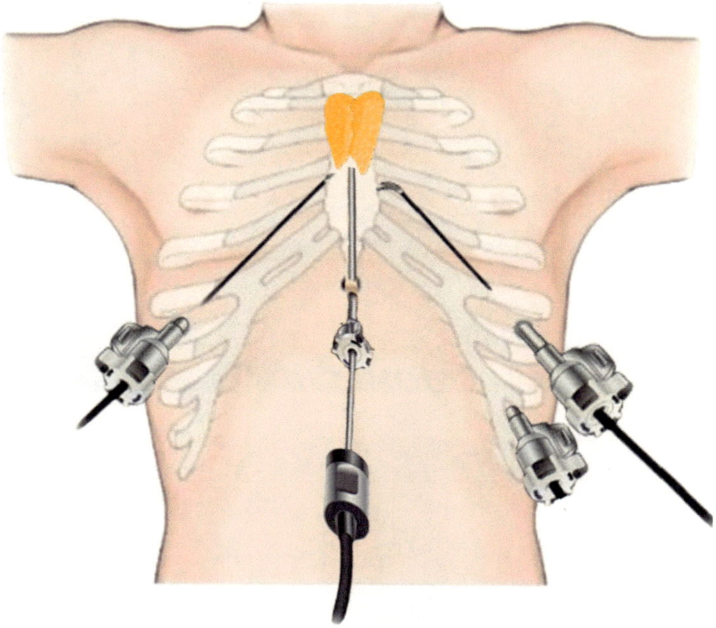

(b) Second, subxiphoid docking

Figure 1.
Positioning and placement of robotic ports in Tangpiroontham's double-docking technique. (a) Initial port placement and docking – the thoracoscope is introduced through the left eighth intercostal space at the anterior axillary line, with an additional working port in the left sixth intercostal space at midaxillary line, further subxiphoid port is added after dissection of lower mediastinal area. (b) Second port placement and docking – an additional 8-mm port is placed into the right pleural cavity at sixth intercostal space, anterior axillary line. Note that prior left eighth intercostal port is currently utilized as an assistant port.

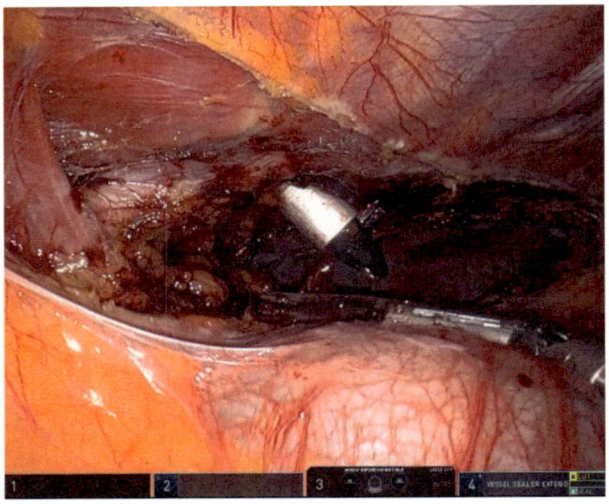

(a)

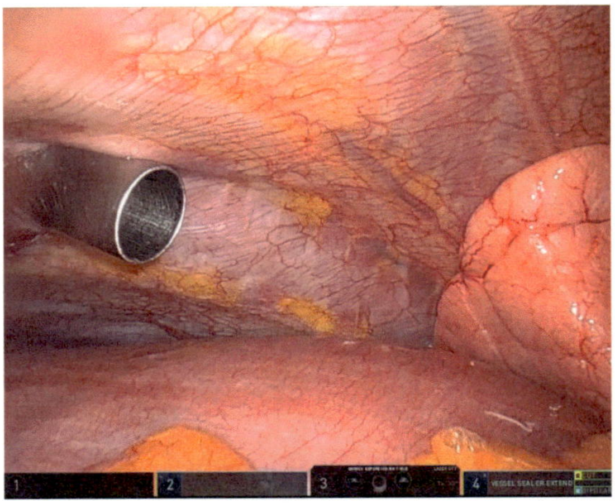

(b)

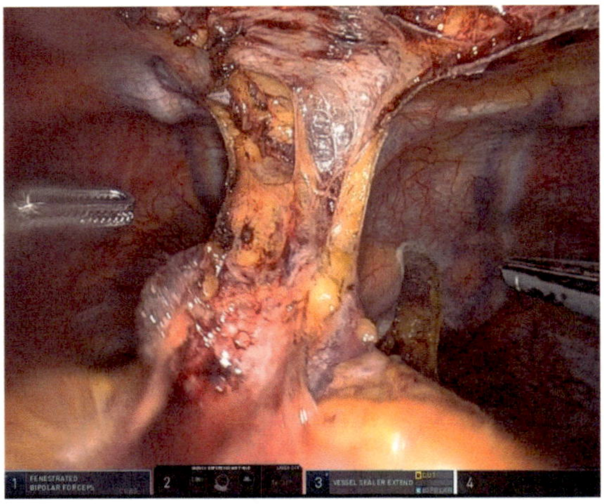

(c)

Figure 2.
Intraoperative images during Tangpiroontham's double-docking technique. (a) Vessel Sealer Extend is used to gently depress the heart during insertion of the subxiphoid port. (b) Intrathoracic view of the right working port at the sixth intercostal space, anterior axillary line. (c) Operative view during the second (subxiphoid) docking is nearly similar to an open sternotomy.

dissected similarly to the left. After both lobes are mobilized, attention turns to the superior horns. Bilateral ventilation can be resumed at this point, as CO_2 insufflation aids in maintaining the operative field. Dissection of the superior poles is performed carefully to avoid injury to the innominate vein and carotid artery. Robotic instruments assist in gentle downward traction of the thymus while the vascular pedicles are clearly visualized, sealed, and divided using the Vessel Sealer (for vessels ≤6–7 mm). Surgical clips may be utilized for larger feeding vessels. The entire thymus and associated fat are placed in an Endobag and retrieved through a lateral port, which can be enlarged if necessary. There is no need to extend the subxiphoid incision in this approach. A single chest drain is positioned on either the left or right side at the port site, preferably on the side where the tumor is dominant. Key operative parison of robotic subxiphoid thymectomy approaches. of this technique is shown in **Table 1**.

Tangpiroontham et al. have demonstrated that this technique is associated with fewer conversions, improved operative times in complex cases, and consistent exposure of bilateral phrenic nerves, particularly in obese patients or those with prior surgical adhesions. While setup time is longer, the benefits in select patient populations make this a valuable technique [6].

3. Comparison between approaches

In comparative analyses, RST has demonstrated several perioperative and functional advantages over other minimally invasive and open approaches. Subxiphoid access provides a midline, symmetrical view of the anterior mediastinum, facilitating simultaneous visualization of both phrenic nerves and superior thymic horns. This contrasts with the lateral transthoracic approach, which often requires partial contralateral dissection under limited visualization,

Steps	Key points
First docking	• Semi-lateral decubitus with the operative side elevated, ipsilateral arm lowered, contralateral arm abducted. • Thoracoscope port at the eighth ICS, anterior axillary line Working port at the sixth ICS, midaxillary line; Vessel Sealer Extend is introduced. • Subxiphoid port; fenestrated bipolar dissector is introduced. • There is no assistant port during the first docking period.
Second docking	• Supine position. • Subxiphoid port becomes a thoracoscopic port. • Prior thoracoscopic port at the sixth ICS becomes a working port. • New contralateral port added at the sixth ICS, midaxillary line, as a working port. Prior assistant port at the eighth ICS becomes an assistant port.
Specimen retrieval	In an Endobag, removed via a lateral port (can be enlarged).
Drain placement	Single chest drain on tumor-dominant side.

Table 1.
Key operative steps: Tangpiroontham double-docking technique.

increasing the technical difficulty of achieving a complete thymectomy in MG or upper pole lesions.

Park et al. conducted a propensity-matched comparison between subxiphoid and lateral RATS, showing significantly shorter chest tube duration (1.4 vs. 2.1 days, $p < 0.05$) and higher postoperative quality-of-life scores in the subxiphoid cohort. In addition, postoperative pain scores were consistently lower in the subxiphoid group at multiple time points, likely due to the avoidance of intercostal nerve compression [7].

Tangpiroontham et al. reported that their double-docking subxiphoid technique further enhanced these benefits, offering improved operative ergonomics, reduced external arm clashing, and consistent bilateral nerve exposure, even in patients with obesity or dense adhesions. Conversion rates to open surgery were lower compared with single-docking and lateral access methods, particularly in complex resections [6].

A meta-analysis pooling subxiphoid versus lateral thymectomy data (both VATS and RATS) found that the subxiphoid approach was associated with reduced intraoperative blood loss, shorter hospital stays, and lower pain scores, alongside superior bilateral phrenic nerve visualization and improved cosmetic outcomes. These findings were consistent across oncologic and MG patient subgroups, suggesting a broad applicability of the subxiphoid route [8].

Lee JH et al. [5] demonstrated in a multi-institutional matched study that uniportal RST using the da Vinci SP system resulted in zero conversions to multiport access (vs. 20% in the uniportal VATS group), shorter drain durations, and reduced hospital stay, while maintaining equivalent pain outcomes. The single midline incision also optimized cosmesis without compromising exposure [5].

In contrast, the lateral RATS approach remains advantageous for selected unilateral lesions, particularly when extensive dissection of contralateral mediastinal fat is not required. Its familiarity to surgeons trained in lateral thoracoscopic approaches and its straightforward port placement make it efficient for smaller, unilateral anterior mediastinal tumors. However, in MG or extended thymectomy cases requiring symmetric bilateral clearance, lateral approaches may be less optimal than subxiphoid access [9].

Overall, the accumulated evidence supports subxiphoid RATS as the preferred minimally invasive approach when complete bilateral mediastinal clearance, reduced intercostal trauma, and superior postoperative recovery are primary goals. The choice between multiportal, uniportal, or double-docking techniques should be individualized based on patient anatomy, disease extent, and surgeon expertise [5–9]. A summarise comparison of robotic subxiphoid thymectomy approaches is demonstrated in **Table 2**.

4. Surgical pitfalls and troubleshooting

In RST, intraoperative pitfalls include limited workspace in patients with elevated BMI, bleeding from the innominate vein or thymic veins, and suboptimal visualization of the contralateral phrenic nerve in inexperienced hands. Managing these challenges requires adequate retrosternal dissection and proper CO_2 insufflation to maintain space. Bleeding control necessitates pre-emptive identification of vascular anatomy and readiness with suction and clips. Conversion to open surgery is rare but should be anticipated in cases of uncontrolled hemorrhage

Feature	Lateral RATS	Multiportal RATS	Uniportal RATS	da Vinci SP – Uniportal RATS	Tangpiroontham – double docking
Number of robotic arms	3–4	3–4	1	1	2–3 (sequential)
Port placement	ICS (uni/bilateral)	Subxiphoid + bilateral subcostal (± assistant)	Single subxiphoid (glove/commercial port)	Single subxiphoid with SP port	Bilateral eighth ICS, left or right sixth ICS, subxiphoid
Docking	Unilateral	Central	Central	Central SP	lateral → subxiphoid (sequential)
CO_2	Optional (6–12 mmHg)	6–10 mmHg	6–10 mmHg	6–12 mmHg	6–12 mmHg
Visual	Limited contra-lateral phrenic nerve exposure	Excellent midline exposure	Excellent midline exposure	Excellent midline exposure	Excellent midline exposure
Features	Familiar setup, direct ICS access	Early adoption of subxiphoid RATS	No intercostal port	No intercostal port, SP-specific articulating arms	Enhanced exposure, better ergonomics for obese or adhesed cases, and no chance of entering the peritoneal cavity
Cosmetic outcome	Variable (intercostal scars)	Good	Excellent	Excellent	Excellent (small 8-mm at subxiphoid)
Learning curve	Low to moderate	Moderate	Steep (due to crowding)	High (SP-specific skills)	Moderate-advanced
Application	TET, MG (limited extended resection)	TET, MG	Early-stage TET, MG	Early-stage TET, MG	TET, MG, complex anatomy, obesity, redo cases

Table 2.
Comparison of robotic subxiphoid thymectomy approaches.

or dense adhesions. Surgeons should not hesitate to convert to an open approach if patient safety or adequate tumor resection cannot be ensured. The double-docking technique has been particularly helpful in cases with distorted mediastinal anatomy or previous sternotomy [6, 10].

5. Learning curve and training

RST requires a steep learning curve, primarily due to the confined working space, complex docking maneuvers, and delicate anatomical dissection. Evidence suggests that a minimum of 20–30 cases is required to attain procedural proficiency [11]. Simulation-based training, structured proctorship, and cadaveric workshops significantly shorten the learning period. Institutional protocols that emphasize team familiarity with equipment, standardized port placements, and troubleshooting protocols have resulted in lower complication rates and enhanced operative efficiency [12, 13].

6. Postoperative follow-up and imaging

Postoperative care includes pain control, respiratory physiotherapy, and early mobilization. Intercostal drainage is typically removed within 24–48 hours. Follow-up imaging is scheduled at every 3–6 months then annually for thymic carcinoma, and every 6–12 months then annually for thymoma with contrast-enhanced CT to evaluate for recurrence or residual disease [14]. Serum acetylcholine receptor antibodies may be monitored in MG patients to assess symptom improvement. The intraoperative use of ICG fluorescence imaging and 3D CT models has been shown to enhance anatomical localization and postoperative assessment accuracy [15].

7. Conclusion

The subxiphoid robotic thymectomy provides a median sternotomy-like operative view, allowing the surgeon to clearly visualize both phrenic nerves and the upper thymic poles. This broad midline perspective facilitates a more complete extended thymectomy. The multiportal and uniportal techniques each offer unique advantages, with emerging modifications such as double docking further optimizing access in a variety of cases.

By avoiding multiple intercostal ports, this approach also minimizes intercostal nerve and vessel injury. Notably, it has proven feasible even in obese patients, with no increase in complications observed in high-BMI cohorts. Comparative studies and meta-analyses consistently report favorable outcomes with subxiphoid thymectomy – including shorter hospital stays and chest tube duration, fewer postoperative complications, and no compromise in oncologic completeness – when compared to lateral VATS or open thymectomy. Conversion rates to open surgery are low, and the ability to extract the specimen through a subxiphoid incision permits removal of large tumors without enlarging intercostal wounds.

Given these advantages – improved bilateral nerve visualization, reduced surgical trauma, better ergonomics, and excellent clinical outcomes – the subxiphoid robotic approach is increasingly being favored over lateral or open techniques, particularly for MG patients, those requiring extensive resections, obese individuals, and others with challenging mediastinal anatomy. This emerging approach emphasizes the oncologic thoroughness of a midline view with the benefits of minimal invasiveness, making it a compelling new standard for thymectomy.

Acknowledgment

The author acknowledges the use of ChatGPT for language polishing in the manuscript.

DOI: http://dx.doi.org/10.5772/intechopen.1013245

Author details

Padungkiat Tangpiroontham* and Krit Vikan
Bangkok Hospital Headquarters, Bangkok, Thailand

*Address all correspondence to: dr.padungkiat@gmail.com

References

[1] Suda T, Kaneda S, Hachimaru A, Tochii D, Maeda R, Tochii S, Takagi Y. Thymectomy via a subxiphoid approach: single-port and robot-assisted. Journal of Thoracic Disease. 2016;**8**(Suppl 3):S265–71. DOI: 10.3978/j.issn.2072-1439.2016.02.34

[2] Zhang H, Chen L, Zheng Y, Wang Z, Geng Y, Wang F, Liu D, He A, Li J, Wang Y. Robot-assisted thymectomy via subxiphoid approach: technical details and early outcomes. Journal of Thoracic Disease. 2018;**10**(3):1677–1682. DOI: 10.21037/jtd.2018.03.07

[3] Chao YK. Refining Subxiphoid Thymectomy: Transitioning from da Vinci Xi to SP Platform. Journal of Chest Surgery. 2025;**58**(1):S9

[4] Lee JH, Hwang J, Park TH, Gu BM, Jung Y, Yi E, Lee S, Hwang SY, Chung JH, Kim HK. Subxiphoid Single-Port Robotic Thymectomy Using the Single-Port Robotic System versus VATS: A Multi-Institutional, Retrospective, and Propensity Score-Matched Study. Cancers(Basel). 2024;**16**(16):2856

[5] Tangpiroontham P. Robotic-Assisted Subxiphoid Thymectomy: Double Docking Technique. 2024. DOI: 10.25373/ctsnet.27161742

[6] Park JH, Kwon Joong N, Kang CH, Park S. In Kyu Park, Young Tae Kim. Robotic subxiphoid thymectomy versus lateral thymectomy: a propensity score-matched comparison. European Journal of Cardio-Thoracic Surgery. 2022;**62**(1): ezac288. DOI: 10.1093/ejcts/ezac288

[7] Li J, Qi G, Liu Y, et al. Meta-analysis of subxiphoid approach versus lateral approach for thoracoscopic Thymectomy. Journal of Cardiothoracic Surgery. 2020;**15**(89). DOI: 10.1186/s13019-020-01135-w

[8] Bae YH, Lee YM, Kim IH, Choi S, Kim HR, Kim YH, Kim DK, Park SI, Yun JK, Lee GD. Comparison of Short-Term Surgical Outcomes for Thymectomy With Various Minimally Invasive Approaches: A Single-Centre Experience. European Journal of Cardio-Thoracic Surgery. 2025;**67**(11): ezaf366. DOI: 10.1093/ejcts/ezaf366

[9] Terra RM, Milanez-de-Campos JR, Haddad R, Trindade JRM, Lauricella LL, Bibas BJ, Pêgo-Fernandes PM. Robotic thoracic surgery for resection of thymoma and tumors of the thymus: technical development and initial experience. Jornal Brasileiro de Pneumologia. 2019;**46**(1):e20180315. DOI: 10.1590/1806-3713/e20180315

[10] Meacci E, Nachira D, Congedo MT, Petracca-Ciavarella L, Vita ML, Porziella V, Chiappetta M, Lococo F, Tabacco D, Triumbari EKA, Margaritora S. Learning Curve of Robot-Assisted Thymectomy: Single Surgeon's 7-Year Experience. Frontiers in Surgery. 2022;**9**:860899. DOI: 10.3389/fsurg.2022.860899

[11] Shahin GMM, Brandon Bravo Bruinsma GJ, Stamenkovic S, Cuesta MA. Training in robotic thoracic surgery-the European way. Annals of Cardiothoracic Surgery. 2019;**8**(2):202–209. DOI: 10.21037/acs.2018.11.06

[12] Deen S, Farivar AS, Louie BE. Thoracic techniques: robotic thymectomy for thymoma. Indian

Journal of Surgical Oncology. 2013;**4**(2):132–7. DOI: 10.1007/s13193-013-0211-5

[13] Wagner OJ, Louie BE, Vallières E, Aye RW, Farivar AS. Near-infrared fluorescence imaging can help identify the contralateral phrenic nerve during robotic thymectomy. Annals of Thoracic Surgery. 2012;**94**(2):622–5. DOI: 10.1016/j.athoracsur.2012.04.119

[14] Zhu L, Zhang L, Zuo C, et al. Long-term outcomes of robot versus video-assisted thymectomy for thymic epithelial tumors: a propensity matched analysis. BMC Surgery. 2024;**24**:365

[15] Choe G, Elmadhun N. Surveillance of thymic epithelial tumors (TETs)-a narrative review. Mediastinum. 2025;**9**:18. DOI: 10.21037/med-25-20